Contents

Contents   vii

List of Figures   xi

List of Tables   xiv

Abbreviations   xvii

1   Introduction   1
    1.1   Background and Significance   1
          1.1.1   Diabetes and It's Complications   1
          1.1.2   Retinal Structure and Function   4
          1.1.3   Diabetic Retinopathy and Public Health   5
          1.1.4   Screening for Diabetic Retinopathy   7
    1.2   Motivation   8
    1.3   Problem Definition   9
    1.4   Research Objectives   9
    1.5   Summary of Contributions   10
    1.6   Organization of Thesis   12
    1.7   Chapter Summary   13

2   Literature Review   14
    2.1   Contribution of Image Processing to Retinal Image Analysis . . .   14

      2.1.1   Exudate Detection 16

      2.1.2   Microaneurysms Detection 16

      2.1.3   Retinal Vessel Segmentation 19

  2.2   Publicly Available Retinal Image Databases 22

  2.3   Chapter Summary 24

3 A K-means clustering approach for exudate detection   25

  3.1   Introduction 25

  3.2   Related Work 25

  3.3   Proposed Method 27

      3.3.1   Optic Disk detection 27

      3.3.2   Feature selection 30

      3.3.3   Coarse segmentation of exudate using K means clustering algorithm 32

      3.3.4   Fine segmentation of exudates by morphological reconstruction 34

  3.4   Results & Discussion 35

      3.4.1   Material 35

      3.4.2   Evaluation 36

      3.4.3   Discussion 37

  3.5   Chapter Summary 39

4 Retinal microaneurysm detection using moment invariant features   41

  4.1   Introduction 41

  4.2   Related Work 42

  4.3   Proposed Method 42

      4.3.1   Pre-processing 43

      4.3.2   Candidate Extraction 44

      4.3.3   Feature Extraction 46

            4.3.3.1   Moment invariant based features 48

            4.3.3.2   Zernike Moments 49

            4.3.3.3   Shape and Intensity based features 52

      4.3.4   RUSBoost Classifier 53

  4.4   Results & Discussion 56

      4.4.1   Material 56

      4.4.2   Evaluation 56

      4.4.3   Discussion 58

  4.5   Chapter Summary 59

5 Retinal vessel segmentation using EFMMNN classifier   63

  5.1   Introduction 63

  5.2   Related Work 64

5.3 Proposed Method 65
   5.3.1 Feature Extraction 66
      5.3.1.1 Difference of Gaussian 66
      5.3.1.2 Phase Stretch Transform 67
      5.3.1.3 Phase Congruency 68
      5.3.1.4 Frangi filter 68
      5.3.1.5 Gabor filter 69
      5.3.1.6 Black Top-Hat Transformation 70
5.4 Classification 71
   5.4.1 Enhanced Fuzzy Min-Max Neural Network 71
      5.4.1.1 Hyperbox Expansion 74
      5.4.1.2 Hyperbox Overlap Test 75
      5.4.1.3 Hyperbox Contraction 76
5.5 Results & Discussion 79
   5.5.1 Material 79
   5.5.2 Parameter Settings 80
   5.5.3 Evaluation 81
   5.5.4 Discussion 82
5.6 Chapter Summary 83

6 Exploiting transfer learning using CBAM-U-Net for efficient retinal vessel segmentation **89**
6.1 Introduction 89
6.2 Related Work 90
6.3 Methodology 91
   6.3.1 Dataset Preparation 91
   6.3.2 CBAM-U-Net 92
      6.3.2.1 Basic U-Net 93
      6.3.2.2 Convolutional Block Attention Module 94
   6.3.3 Transfer Learning 96
   6.3.4 Performance Evaluation Metrics 98
6.4 Results & Discussion 99
   6.4.1 Comparison against transfer learning 99
   6.4.2 Comparison against existing DL methods 102
6.5 Conclusion 102
6.6 Chapter Summary 104

7 Conclusion and Future Scope **113**
7.1 Conclusion 113
   7.1.1 Exudate Detection 114
   7.1.2 MA Detection 114
   7.1.3 Vessel Segmentation 115

7.2   Future Research Direction 116

Bibliography   **117**

List of Figures

1.1 Estimated number of people with diabetes per region worldwide in 2019 and 2045 (Image source: IDF Atlas 2019). 2

1.2 Diabetes complications (Image source: The Diabetes Centre). . . . 3

1.3 (a) Anatomy of Eye and (b) Retinal Fundus Image 5

1.4 Clinical signs of DR 6

1.5 Stages of DR: (a) NPDR and (b) PDR 6

3.1 Retina Image containing Exudates 26

3.2 Morphological reconstruction by Dilation 28

3.3 Steps in OD Detection 30

3.4 Feature selected for K-means clustering 31

3.5 Clusters obtained after K-means Clustering 33

3.6 Steps in exudate detection 35

3.7 ROC Curve for the exudate detection on DIARETDB1 database . . . 37

3.8 Sample images of DIARETDB1 database illustrating the OD and exudate detection using proposed method 39

3.9 Sample images of DRISHTI database illustrating the OD and exudate detection using proposed method 40

4.1 Retinal Fundus Image containing Microaneurysm 42

4.2 Block Diagram of the proposed approach for MA detection 43

4.3 Steps for Candidate Segmentation (a) RGB Image from ROC Dataset (b) Pre-processed Image (c) Candidate Extraction 46

4.4 (a) Eight group of pixels are marked with white circular candidate regions Ak and Bk with k = 1,2,3,4; Ak are microaneurysm pixels whereas Bk are spurious pixels. (b)-(d) are zoomed sub-images of extracted MA pixels, (e)-(g) are zoomed sub-images of extracted spurious objects 50

4.5 (a) $M \times M$ size candidate (ROI) with function $c(x, y)$ and (b) function $c(x, y)$ mapped onto unit circle. 51

4.6 FROC curve analysis of proposed approach on ROC, DIARETDB1 and e-ophtha dataset Note: x-axis scale is logarithmic 57

4.7 FROC curve analysis for different class-imbalance approaches in MA detection on ROC dataset 59

4.8 FROC curve analysis for different class-imbalance approaches in MA detection on DIARETDB1 dataset 61

4.9 FROC curve analysis for different class-imbalance approaches in MA detection on e-ophtha dataset 61

5.1 Schematic Diagram of proposed method for retinal vessel segmentation 65

5.2 (a) Gray Scale Image; Illustration of extracted features for vessel segmentation: (b) Difference of Gaussian, (c) Phase Stretch Transform, (d) Phase Congruency, (e) Frangi filtering, (f) Gabor filtering 71

5.3 Features extracted using black top-hat transformation at different scales 72

5.4 EFMMNN for the proposed method 74

5.5 Results of proposed vessel segmentation on random images of DRIVE dataset: Column-wise (a) RGB Image, (b) Groundtruth Image, (c) Proposed vessel segmentation output Image 87

5.6 Results of proposed vessel segmentation on random images of STARE dataset : Column-wise (a) RGB Image, (b) Groundtruth Image, (c) Proposed vessel segmentation output Image 88

6.1 CBAM-U-Net architecture with image input tile of size 64×64 . . . 93

6.2 Convolutional Block Attention Module (CBAM) 94

6.3 Individual Channel-attention module & Spatial-attention module . 96

6.4 (a) 64×64 size training patches given as input to the CBAM-U-Net (b) Patches from the corresponding groundtruth 100

6.5 Comparison of training from scratch and training using pre-trained weights on (a) STARE (b) CHASE (c) HRF dataset 101

6.6 ROC Curve for the proposed network for (a) DRIVE dataset (b) STARE dataset (with TL) (c) CHASE dataset (with TL) (d) HRF dataset (with TL) 103

6.7 Column-wise: 1st Column : Randomly extracted patches from retinal images showcasing various challenging scenarios ; 2nd Column : Groundtruth for the corresponding input patches ; 3rd Column : Output of the proposed algorithm for the corresponding patches . . 107

6.8 Column-wise: 1st Column : Randomly selected images from DRIVE dataset ; 2nd Column : Groundtruth for the corresponding input images ; 3rd Column : Output of the proposed algorithm for the corresponding images 109

6.9 Column-wise: 1st Column : Randomly selected images from STARE dataset ; 2nd Column : Groundtruth for the corresponding input images ; 3rd Column : Output of the proposed algorithm for the corresponding images 110

6.10 Column-wise: 1st Column : Randomly selected images from CHASE dataset ; 2nd Column : Groundtruth for the corresponding input images ; 3rd Column : Output of the proposed algorithm for the corresponding images 111

6.11 Column-wise: 1st Column : Randomly selected images from HRF dataset ; 2nd Column : Groundtruth for the corresponding input images ; 3rd Column : Output of the proposed algorithm for the corresponding images 112

List of Tables

1.1   International clinical DR severity scale   7

3.1   DIARETDB1 results for proposed method for exudate detection   . .   37

3.2   Comparison of state-of-the-art exudate detection method for DI-ARETDB1 Database   38

4.1   Module of the logarithm of invariant moments $\phi_1 - \phi_4$ calculated from the marked circular candidate regions show in Figure 4.4(a).   49

4.2   Description of features extracted for each candidate region in MA classification   53

4.3   Comparison of state-of-the-art MA detection methods at predefined FPI for ROC dataset   60

4.4   Comparison of state-of-the-art MA detection methods at predefined FPI for DIARETDB1 dataset   60

4.5   Comparison of state-of-the-art MA detection methods at predefined FPI for e-ophtha dataset   60

4.6   Row-wise: (a) Retinal RGB Fundus Image (b) Groundtruth Image for the RGB image of respective column (c) Final Output Image after classification stage.   62

5.1   No. of hyperboxes obtained w.r.t. Θ   79

5.2   Parameter values used during the proposed approach   81

5.3   Classification measure   81

5.4   Confusion matrix for DRIVE dataset   82

5.5   Confusion matrix for STARE dataset   82

5.6   Performance measure   82

5.7   Individual imagewise result on DRIVE dataset   84

5.8   Individual imagewise result on STARE dataset   85

5.9   Comparative analysis of the supervised learning based state-of-the-art methods on DRIVE dataset   86

5.10   Comparative analysis of the supervised learning based state-of-the-art methods on STARE dataset   86

6.1   Publicly available datasets used in the proposed approach   105

6.2 Comparison of performance metrics of proposed network on training with scratch and training using transfer learning 106

6.3 Comparative analysis of state-of-the-art deep learning approaches on different datasets 108

List of Algorithms

4.1   Algorithm depicting the steps in candidate extraction for MA detection **47**

4.2   Pseudocode for RUSBoost classifier **55**

5.1   Pseudocode for EFMMNN Classifier **78**

Abbreviations

ANN	Artificial Neural Network
CAD	Computer Aided Diagnosis
CLAHE	Contrast Limited Adaptive Histogram Equalization
CBAM	Convolutional Block Attention Module
CNN	Convolutional Neural Network
DL	Deep Learning
DR	Diabetic Retinopathy
DoG	Difference of Gaussian
EFMMNN	Enhanced Fuzzy Min Max Neural Network
EX	Hard Exudates
FOV	Field of Vision
FROC	Free Response Operating Characteristic
HE	Haemorrhages
ICO	International Council of Ophthalmology
IDF	International Diabetes Federation
k-NN	k Nearest Neighbour
MA	Microaneurysms
NPDR	Non Proliferative Diabetic Retinopathy
OD	Optic Disk
PCA	Principle Component Analysis
PDR	Proliferative Diabetic Retinopathy
PST	Phase Stretch Transform

ROC	Receiver Operating Characteristic
RUS	Random Undersampling
TL	Transfer Learning
SE	Soft Exudates

Chapter 1

Introduction

1.1 Background and Significance

1.1.1 Diabetes and It's Complications

Diabetes is a metabolic disorder, characterized by uncontrolled blood sugar levels in the blood. Diabetes is an outcome of either pancreas not producing enough insulin or not utilizing the produced hormone effectively [1]. The carbohydrates in the food we eat are broken down to glucose, and insulin is the hormone responsible to take in the glucose to be used for energy. If the required energy is suffice, insulin signals the liver to store the glucose as glycogen. Insulin maintains a balance between the high (hyperglycaemia) and low (hypoglycaemia) sugar levels. There are three categories of Diabetes:

- Type-I Diabetes : The Islets of Langherhans i.e β cells in pancreas are destroyed by body's autoimmune system, resulting in failure of insulin production in human body.

- Type-II Diabetes : The body provides resistance to insulin or the pancreas secret insufficient insulin, resulting in lack of required insulin in human body.

- Gestational diabetes : This is observed in pregnant women when body is not able to produce extra insulin needed during pregnancy. Generally, it gets resolved after the baby's birth.

Insulin insufficiency is the prime reason of diabetes. The reason for attack of body's auto-immune system on pancreas in Type-I diabetes is unknown but the reason for ever increasing Type-II diabetes population is lifestyle of people which includes insufficient physical activity, high-calorie diet resulting into obesity & high blood pressure which facilitate insulin resistance in body. Uncontrolled Diabetes brings too many complications along with it. Thus, the Diabetes has become the leading health emergency across the world.

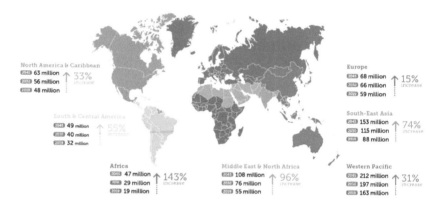

FIGURE 1.1: Estimated number of people with diabetes per region worldwide in 2019 and 2045 (Image source: IDF Atlas 2019).

According to IDF Atlas 2019 [2], approximately 463 million working age population (20-79 years) are having diabetes. This is estimated to rise to 700 million by 2045 (Figure 1.1). Diabetes is one of the most rapidly growing health issues of the 21st century, and has more than tripled the number of adults with diabetes in the past 20 years. Every 6 seconds someone in the world is diagnosed with diabetes. The more important fact to mention is the countries like China (116.4 million) and India (77 million) have majority of population with diabetes. As the prevalence of diabetes is rising worldwide, so are its complications. Diabetes increase the risk of long-term complications, major related to damage of blood vessels. The primary complication amongst it is damage to blood vessels of eyes, kidney and nerves leading to retinopathy, nephropathy and neuropathy respectively. Hyperglycaemia also leads to other health issues like heart disease or stroke, peripheral vascular disease, diabetic foot amputation, osteoporosis and many more. Figure 1.2 illustrates the complications of diabetes on different organs.

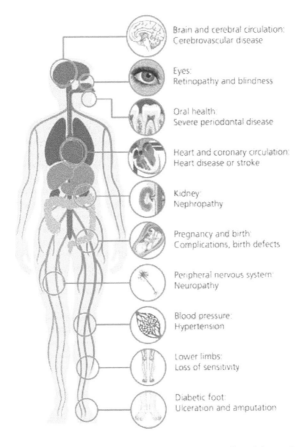

Brain and cerebral circulation:
Cerebrovascular disease

Eyes:
Retinopathy and blindness

Oral health:
Severe periodontal disease

Heart and coronary circulation:
Heart disease or stroke

Kidney:
Nephropathy

Pregnancy and birth:
Complications, birth defects

Peripheral nervous system:
Neuropathy

Blood pressure:
Hypertension

Lower limbs:
Loss of sensitivity

Diabetic foot:
Ulceration and amputation

FIGURE 1.2: Diabetes complications (Image source: The Diabetes Centre).

Diabetic eye disease is a serious complication of diabetes, comprising preponderantly of Diabetic Retinopathy (DR). DR occurs as a direct outcome of chronic hyperglycaemia, causing damage to blood retinal barrier, leading to leakage and blockage in retinal capillaries [3]. This may cause loss of vision and sooner or later lead to blindness. DR is recognised as one of the leading causes of impaired vision with severe personal and socio-economic implications in working age population, inspite of being possibly preventable and treatable. DR affects about one out of three diabetic patients. The span of diabetes is the most effective predictor of DR prevalence. According to IDF, it is estimated that about 191 million diabetic people are likely to develop DR by 2030. Current estimates show 56.3 million people worsening to vision-threatening DR if immediate and proper steps are not taken. Early diagnosis and timely medical intervention of DR can prevent vision impairment and blindness. Regular eye screening should therefore be an essential component of routine diabetes care provided by primary healthcare professionals. However, geographical conditions and inadequate resources make regular eye examination difficult in many countries. Given the overview of diabetes and its impact on human body, this chapter focusses on definition and classification of DR, motivation, research objective and need for computer-aided screening of DR.

1.1.2 Retinal Structure and Function

Human eye is the spherical organ responsible for our vision. It has an approximate sagittal diameter of 24 to 25 mm and transverse diameter of 24 mm. Eye consist of number of components as shown in Figure 1.3, which perform their respective functions and collectively responsible to create the vision. Light enters the eye through pupil and the appropriate amount of it is directed towards the lens with the help of iris and cornea.

The lens refracts the light onto the retina. Retina is a light sensitive layer that forms the back lining of eye. Photoreceptor cells in retina senses light and creates electrical impulses that travel through the optic nerve to the brain. These signals are further converted into images and visual perceptions in the visual cortex of brain. There are two photoreceptor cells - rods and cones. Rods detect motion and functions best in dim light. Cones are responsible for colour vision and performs best in bright light. The central area of retina has a yellow spot called macula. A small depression at the centre of macula, responsible for maximum visual acuity is fovea. A blind spot on the retina is called as optic disk, which is entry point of the main blood vessels that supply nourishment to retina.

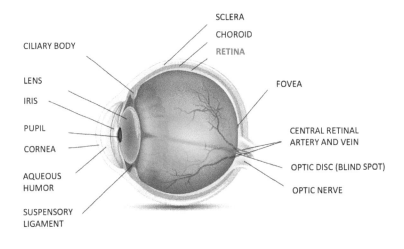

(a)

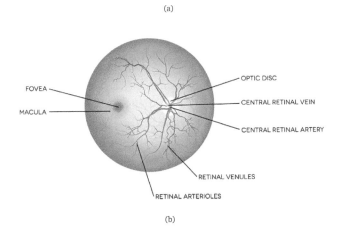

(b)

FIGURE 1.3: (a) Anatomy of Eye and (b) Retinal Fundus Image

1.1.3 Diabetic Retinopathy and Public Health

Diabetic Retinopathy (DR) is an outcome of prolonged diabetes which directly or indirectly affect the human vision. DR is asymptomatic in its early stages and the late diagnosis lead to undeviating loss of vision. International Council of Ophthalmology (ICO) guidelines show that 1 in 3 individual with diabetes had some form of DR and also noted that 1 in 10 had vision threatening DR [4].

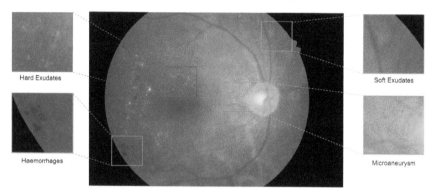

FIGURE 1.4: Clinical signs of DR

DR primarily happens in one of the two phases known as non-proliferative diabetic retinopathy (NPDR) and proliferative diabetic retinopathy (PDR) as shown in Figure 1.5. The presence of one or more retinal lesions like microaneurysms (MA), haemorrhages (HE), hard exudates (EX), soft exudates (SE) is categorized as NPDR [5]. The venous beading or retinal detachment i.e. neovascularization along with the presence of above findings are classified as PDR. The International Clinical DR severity scales [6] given in Table 1.1 provides a unified concord for the necessary screening and treatment of DR.

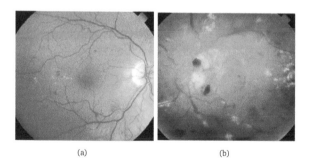

(a)   (b)

FIGURE 1.5: Stages of DR: (a) NPDR and (b) PDR

TABLE 1.1: International clinical DR severity scale

Disease Severity Level	Findings
No apparent retinopathy	No visible sign of abnormalities
Mild NPDR	Only presence of MAs
Moderate NPDR	More than just MAs but less than severe NPDR
Severe NPDR	Moderate NPDR and any of the following: • > 20 intraretinal HEs (each quadrant) • Venous beading (in $\geq$ 2 quadrants) • Intraretinal microvascular abnormalities (in $\geq$ 1 quadrant) • no signs of PDR
PDR	Severe NPDR and one or both of the following: • Neovascularization • Vitreous/preretinal HE

1.1.4 Screening for Diabetic Retinopathy

DR perceive no symptoms until the late progression of the disease which could lead to visual impairment or irreparable loss. Early screening and the required treatment (if any) is essential for the patients prone to have this disease. Regular and timely check-up of retina is prescribed to diabetic patients for early monitoring of DR. The recent time screening of retina with the help of non-mydriatic digital retinal fundus camera is non-invasive and cost-effective. The operation of this camera requires just a basic training in comparison with the other techniques like indirect ophthalmoscopy and slit-lamp fundus bio-microscopy which need dilated pupils as well as expertise for its operation. Fundus imaging is preferred way of screening DR as it comes with several advantages. The awareness of the DR progression and better understanding of consequences is must for its management and early treatment.

The timely screening and necessary preventive measures for DR mainly depend on the accessibility of the efficient clinicians and supporting health care facilities. India has population ratio of 1:107,000 against a national ophthalmologist, which vary as 1:9000 in some region and as 1:608,000 in some other regions [7]. This wide variation and its management to reach out the probable population of DR for screening is a matter of concern worldwide. The mass screening DR workshop with the help of eye care experts can assist in reaching out huge population and their timely examination. The purpose of the screening program is to iden-tify patients who may need retinal specialist therapy and other patients who may simply have regular biannual or annual screening. The success of screening work-shops depends on the screened attendees, the cost involved and the efficiency of screening method with reference to sensitivity and specificity. Computer aided di-agnosis (CAD) with the help of advanced machine learning and computer vision algorithms assists the retinal care experts in speedy, cost-effective and efficient di-agnosis. Thus, the research in computer aided medical imaging is booming with a motive to aid the clinical health experts in easy and efficient screening of anoma-lies, especially during the mass screening programs.

1.2   Motivation

Diabetic Retinopathy (DR) is the result of prolonged effect of diabetes on the retina. The disease show no prominent symptoms in its initial stages and late intervention could lead to visual impairment. Diabetes is one of the fastest grow-ing health issue globally and brings it several complications along.

The motivation behind this thesis are the people suffering with diabetes. Type-II Diabetes is the outcome of lifestyle of an individual but Type-I Diabetes occuring in children is a metabolic disorder. The prime motivation behind this work of Dia-betic Retinopathy are the children suffering with Type-I Diabetes including myself. I am Type-I Diabetic since the age of 10 and dependant on insulin. Inspite of strin-gent control, I have been diagnosed with tiny microaneurysms in my left retina. Thus, work is dedicated to such children and aims to add few drops to this wide ocean of research ongoing in screening of DR.

A timely screening of retina should be an essential part of the routine of diabetic patients. The conventional approaches of DR screening are time consuming, ex-pensive and could be sometimes prone to error. Thus, computer aided screening of DR using emerging computer vision and machine learning techniques is proving to be of great help to meet the requirements of clinical practice. This ensures cost efficient, speedy and effective treatment with the assistance of ophthalmologists and clinical experts. The aim of this research is to develop algorithms for com-puter aided diagnosis of several pathologies associated with DR. The validation of algorithms and comparison with the existing literature is done using the publicly available retinal image datasets and their respective ground truth. We have focussed on various issues like retinal vessel segmentation, EX detection and MA detection. These computer aided algorithms can surely assist ophthalmologists for quick, cost-effective and reliable screening of DR.

1.3   Problem Definition

The main objective of the work is to contribute to the computer aided screening and diagnosis of various lesions in DR. The extraction of normal (optic disk (OD) and retinal vessels) and abnormal (MA, HE, EX) retinal structures from the retinal images is the main aim of the research. The novel algorithms could contribute in screening and better diagnosis of the disease and its severity. The automated system can assist ophthalmologists for better interpretation of retinal images. We have focussed on early screening of DR through the various contributions briefed in synopsis. There is no particular link in methodologies opted in each contribution but they are linked through screening of the disease DR. The proposed approaches attempts to extract the retinal features which are mandate during the automated retinal image analysis for DR screening.

1.4   Research Objectives

1. Study of state-of-the-art methods and finding out the potential research problems for effective screening of DR.

2. Development of methods for the segmentation of retinal vessels which is the pre-requisite during each stage of DR screening.

3. Development of algorithm for detection of microaneurysms (MA) to diagnose DR in its early stages.

4. Development of algorithm for detection of exudates (EX) for the screening of DR.

1.5 Summary of Contributions

1. A K-means clustering approach for exudate detection

   EX are prominent sign of NPDR which is the crucial cause of loss of sight in patients suffering with diabetes. Early diagnosis of the disease through automated screening and prompt treatment has proven beneficial in preventing the spread of disease and irreparable visual impairment. This contribution is an attempt to help the ophthalmologists in the screening process of DR to detect EX from non-mydriatic low-contrast retinal digital images faster and more easily. This contribution proposes a method using K-means clustering and morphological image processing for detection of EX. The OD might get misdiagnosed as EX area due to nearly same contrast as like the EX, so the OD area is eliminated from the retinal images to avoid its intervention in EX detection. The publicly available retinal images of DIARETDB1 database along with expert ophthalmologist's hand-drawn groundtruth images are used to validate the proposed approach.

2. Retinal microaneurysm detection using moment invariant features

   The first clinically observable lesion on retina is microaneurysm (MA). Thus, the screening of MA is an earliest measure to screen and treat DR. Thus the proposed contribution aims to automatically segment MA from fundus images for an early and easy screening of DR. By the virtue of modern computer vision techniques, it aims to assist ophthalmologists in early screening of DR, especially during mass screening workshops. A 16 characteristic feature vector extracted from moment invariants along with shape and intensity based features is given to RUSBoosted tree classifier to classify true MA from non-MA candidates. Invariant moment features are demonstrated as excellent MA shape descriptor along with shape and intensity features. Random undersampling adaboost classifier is employed to classify minority MA from spurious candidates. The proposed approach is evaluated on publicly available DIARETDB1, ROC and e-ophtha datasets. The experimental results and performance of the proposed method evidences its ability and strong candidature for use in real time screening and diagnosis of DR.

3. Retinal Vessel Segmentation using enhanced fuzzy min-max neural network

Automated segmentation of retinal vessels plays a pivotal role in early diagnosis of ophthalmic disorders. Retinal vessel segmentation is often a prerequisite in PDR treatment and image registration. A blood vessel segmentation algorithm using an enhanced fuzzy min-max neural network (EFMMNN) supervised classifier is proposed in this contribution. An optimal 11-D feature vector consisting of spatial as well as frequency domain features extracted from each pixel of a fundus image is input to the neural network. The essence of the method is its hyperbox classifier which performs online learning and gives binary output without any need of post-processing. A three layered neural network without any need of back propagation algorithm outperforms the other existing supervised classification methods. The method is tested on publicly available databases DRIVE and STARE. The proposed method exhibits efficient performance and can be implemented in CAD of retinal diseases.

4. Exploiting transfer learning using CBAM-U-Net for efficient retinal vessel segmentation

Deep learning (DL) architectures are achieving the state-of-the-art performances in medical image segmentation. Thus, we have explored a semantic segmentation based CBAM-U-Net to segment the retinal vessels in this contribution. Convolutional block attention module (CBAM) is included at bottleneck of U-Net and achieves the better results than existing DL network architectures utilized for retinal vessel segmentation. Further, we exploit the concept of transfer learning and showcase its importance in increasing accuracy of retinal vessel segmentation. The CBAM-U-Net is trained on the publicly available DRIVE dataset and this knowledge of pre-trained network is used for training the network on different retinal image datasets. As the network need not be trained from scratch for these datasets, it attains the higher accuracies in lesser training time and less number of epochs. The transfer learning approach is validated on STARE, CHASE-DB1 and HRF datasets. The proposed algorithm excels in its performance as compared to the state-of-the-art techniques and the exploration of transfer learning for vessel segmentation provides new ways for efficient retinal image analysis.

1.6   Organization of Thesis

This thesis is organized in seven different chapters. This chapter has presented the motivation behind the research involved in this thesis, the objectives and its main contributions. In addition, it also introduces the thesis outline.

Chapter 2 introduces the existing state-of-the-art techniques for computer aided screening of DR. The chapter briefs the literature for retinal vessel segmentation, EX detection and MA detection in three different sections respectively. The chapter also introduces the publicly available datasets for research in automated diagnosis of several lesions associated with DR.

Chapter 3 proposes a EX detection method using K-means clustering and morphological image processing The OD is also detected & eliminated from the retinal images to avoid its intervention in EX detection. This algorithm is an attempt to help the ophthalmologists to detect EX from non-mydriatic low-contrast retinal digital images faster and more easily.

Chapter 4 focuses to segment MA from fundus images for an early and easy screening of DR. A 16 characteristic feature vector extracted from moment invariants along with shape and intensity based features is given to RUSBoosted tree classifier to detect minority class MA from spurious candidates. RUSBoosted classifier deals with the issue of class imbalance.

Chapter 5 presents a novel approach to extract the retinal vessels from a retinal fundus image. The approach involves the use of EFMMNN which employs a hyper-box classifier to differentiate between vessel and non-vessel pixels. The algorithm is validated using publicly available datasets and its performance makes it suitable for use in CAD of DR.

Chapter 6 explores the DL architecture in combination with the transfer learning. An attention module based U-Net is utilised for segmenting retinal vessels. Further, the use of pre-trained weights is employed in training the network with different retinal datasets which result in improved performance of vessel segmentation. The phenomenon of transfer learning is explored in retina image analysis

Chapter 7 concludes the thesis with the brief summary of contributions, limitations of work and discussion on the future scope.

1.7 Chapter Summary

The chapter is a summary to basic and biological information of DR needed to understand the medical terms used during the thesis. The chapter presents a brief to Diabetes and its related complications, DR, its global prevalence and socio-economic burden. Further, it introduces structure of retina and its functions. The grading and various stages involved in progression of DR are also discussed. Thereafter, the importance of DR screening and the need for CAD of DR instead of manual time-consuming procedure is elaborated. The recent machine learning and computer vision techniques along with advance medical imaging equipment can assist the ophthalmologists and health care workers in automated CAD of DR. The motivation and research objective of thesis are also summarized in the chapter. The next chapter provides a literature survey to various pathologies and retinal vessel segmentation involved in screening of DR.

Chapter 2

Literature Review

2.1 Contribution of Image Processing to Retinal Image Analysis

DR comprises of several lesion categories like microaneurysms (MA), haemorrhages (HE), hard exudates (EX), soft exudates (SE). The detection of retinal structures like optic disk (OD), fovea, retinal vessels is also a pre-requisite during the automated retinal image analysis. Extensive research have been carried out with the help of modern computer vision and machine learning technologies for the early screening of DR. The state-of-the-art techniques and ongoing rapidly booming research in deep learning (DL) are example of great accomplishments and way to future advancements. The following subsections reveal a brief on the techniques carried out so far in the CAD screening of DR.

Several approaches have been extended as a review to the existing algorithms in computer aided screening of diabetic retinopathy (DR). The general approach for finding out the normal or abnormal structures involves several stages, typically: image preprocessing for contrast enhancement or illumination equalization, candidate segmentation, feature extraction, and classification. The pathogenesis of DR is ornately explained in the research study by Eshaq et al. [8]. Patton et al. [9] also discussed the lesions associated with DR and the initial approaches to detect the retinal structures. Later, the review of literature till year 2008 for automated screening of DR has been reported in [10] by Winder et al. The literature on detection of normal and abnormal structures in retina is categorised in different sections in this review. Some of the review articles [11, 12] emphasises on large scale screening of automated retinal lesion detection along with the review of methods for lesion segmentation. Few approaches [13, 14] focus on feature extraction methods and CAD in the existing literature for DR screening. These techniques features the overall screening outcome with the interdependence of several segments involved in retinal lesion and anatomical structure detection. A recent review article on machine learning methods for retinal vessel segmentation by Mookiah et al [15] provides a detailed summary of key reported algorithms, datasets as well as segmentation challenges in conventional as well as DL techniques.

DL is the representation learning artificial intelligence function based on multi-layered neural networks. Several approaches have been studied for automated retinal image analysis because of its automatic representation learning of intricate features as well as characteristic of preserving local image relations. DL approaches have been extensively studied during a past decade in retinal image analysis by utilizing off-the-shelf convolutional neural network (CNN) features. Several applications involved in DR as like the segmentation of vessels [16], red lesion detection [17, 18], multi-scale shallow CNN for DR grading [19] and the automated screening of DR [20, 21] are presented using CNN and DL. A systematic and meta-analysis based review by Islam et al. [22] on detecting DR reveals the high performance metrics attained from DL algorithms. Some approaches like [23] are trained utilising CNN from scratch whereas others are initialized using the parameters of pre-trained models and then the network is fine-tuned [24]. There has been a noteworthy development in the CAD of DR using CNN architectures in recent times. Similarly, Google Inc. [25] trained a CNN by utilizing a retrospective database of 128,175 images for DR classification. Some hybrid algorithms are trained using multiple semi-dependent CNN's based on the appearance of retinal lesions [26]. A step further, [27] demonstrated an ability of lesion segmentation based on the CNN trained for image level classification. However, Lynch et al. [28] demonstrated that the hybrid algorithms based on multiple semi-dependent ConvNets might offer a more robust option for DR referral screening, stressing the importance of lesion segmentation.

2.1.1 Exudate Detection

Several techniques have been proposed for EX detection including the morphological image processing, supervised and unsupervised way of classification. Walter et al. [29] proposed a method for automated finding of EX in color eye fundus images using mathematical morphology techniques (e.g. morphological reconstruction). Sopharak et al. [30] and Welfer et al. [31] also described a method very similar to the method as proposed in [29]. Sopharak et al. [32] also used fuzzy c-means clustering to coarsely detect EX followed by morphological techniques. However, the limitation of this method is that it produces high false positives. The inverse surface thresholding approach in [33] finds EX with greater performance indices but fixing a threshold is a limitation. The supervised classification method of EX detection using neural networks have been proposed in [34, 35, 36, 37, 38]. The SVM approach in [39], mixture model approach in [40], region growing segmentation algorithm in [41], adaptive fuzzy logic approach in [42] have been also seek to detect EX.

2.1.2 Microaneurysms Detection

The first clinically observable lesion on retina is microaneurysms (MA). Thus, the screening of MA is an earliest measure to screen and treat DR. There has been extensive investigation and research carried out for the extraction of MA and HEM from the retinal images. We have compiled the literature for red lesion detection into a review paper to have quantitative comparison and qualitative findings in state-of-the-art methods and identify the existing gaps.

During the initial phase of research on DR, fluorescein angiograms were used for computer aided MA detection. Angiography being an invasive technique is unsuitable for regular DR screening, thus further RGB fundus images replaced angiograms for DR analysis. Sinthanayothin et al. [41] introduced a new technique 'moat operator' used to sharpen the edges of lesion followed by recursive region growing segmentation and thresholding. Walter et al. [43] employed morphological diameter closing to extract candidates and used kernel density estimation to classify MA. Niemeijer et al. [44] combined the techniques of mathematical morphology and pixel classification for candidate extraction. New features were introduced to the approach proposed by Frame et al. [45] and k-Nearest Neighbour (k-NN) is used for classification. Mizutani et al. [46] employed a double ring filter followed by elimination of blood vessels. The rule based and Artificial Neural Network (ANN) classification technique was used to detect true MAs. Sanchez et al. [47] proposed candidate extraction using mixture model-based clustering and classification by means of logistic regression.

Zhang et al. [48] proposed a new approach to detect coarse candidates by multi-scale correlation filtering and applied rule-based table to classify MAs. The approach is modified in [49] with the use of sparse representation classifier using dictionaries. Quellec et al. [50] used a template matching technique using wavelets to detect MA. The MA are modelled with rotation-symmetric Gaussian function and the best adapted wavelet was found by applying the lifting scheme framework. Ram et al. [51] proposed a method to detect only targeted MA and rejection of false clutters. Shape based features and clutter structures to characterize MA are introduced and target oriented rejection technique is utilized.

Giancardo et al. [52] proposed an approach utilizing radon-based features to identify MA with minimal image processing. A support vector machine (SVM) is used to classify MA. Different pre-processing and candidate extraction techniques are explored in the approached proposed by Antal and Hajdu [53]. An ensemble-based framework is created to find out the best combination. Lazar and Hazdu [54] proposed directional cross section profile analysis followed by a peak detection on each profile to extract the respective statistical and measurement features. These set of descriptors are input for a Bayesian classifier to identify true red lesions.

Akram et al. [55] used Gabor filter banks to extract candidates from pre-processed image. A hybrid classifier comprising of m-mediods based classifier and Gaussian mixture model is used to classify MA from spurious candidates. In approach proposed by Adal et al. [56], candidate regions are modelled as blobs and several robust blob descriptors are proposed. Local scale estimation is used to detect blobs and a semi supervised approach is used for classification. Dai et al. [57] utilized gradient vector analysis for extracting candidates and vessel removal. MA candidates are less in number as compared to non-MA during candidate extraction stage. Thus, a RUSBoost classifier approach is used for identification of true MA which deals with the class imbalance issue.

Seoud et al. [58] introduced new dynamic shape features to characterize red lesions followed by random forest classifier. Shah et al. [59] employed curvelet transform to extract candidates and rule-based classifier to classify MA from non-MA candidates. Wu et al. [60] proposed an approach using profile features similar to method in [54], with additional local, shape and intensity-based features used to detect lesions. Naïve Bayes, k-NN and AdaBoost classifiers are employed in final classification stage. Wang et al. [61] used dark object filtering to locate candidates. Singular spectrum analysis is then employed to cross-section profiles and its correlation coefficient is used to differentiate MA and non-MA profiles. A set of statistical profile features and k-NN classifier were used for final classification of MA.

Kar and Maity [62] obtained maximum matched filter response and Laplacian of Gaussian response through differential evolution algorithm. The maximization of mutual information of these two responses is employed in red lesion detection. Ren et al. [63] employed adaptive SMOTE to deal with class imbalance learning along with ensemble of boosting, bagging and random subspace classifier to improve the MA detection process. The sparse principle component analysis (PCA) based unsupervised classification approach is proposed by Zhou et al. [64] for detecting red lesions. The class imbalance problem is avoided in this approach since it does not require MA training samples. Local convergence index filters are extracted for each candidate and used in feature set along with shape and intensity based features in the approach given by Dashtbozorg et al. [65]. The hybrid undersampling boosting classifier is used to improve the MA detection. Cao et al. [66] analysed MA detection using 25×25 pixel patches of fundus images. The patches were given directly as input to random forest, neural network and support vector machine. PCA and random forest features are explored for input data dimension reduction. Along with statistical features, Deepa et al. [67] employed discrete Stockwell transform to classify MA from non-MA candidates. Derwin et al. [68] used a local neighbourhood differential coherence pattern for feature extraction particularly to capture texture characteristics. This is followed by feed forward neural network for classification.

In recent years, DL is ongoing boom in the area of computer vision and medical image processing. It has gained significant recognition for the DR detection due to ts performance. Few MA detection approaches using DL techniques are explored in [17], [18]. Orlando et al. [17] combined both the CNN learned and hand-crafted features to improve the red lesion detection. This hybrid feature vector is given to random forest classifier to classify true lesions from false positives. Chudzik et al. [18] proposed a novel patch-based CNN with batch normalization and dice coefficient loss function to identify MA. The method also deals with the knowledge transfer amongst small datasets in MA detection.

2.1.3   Retinal Vessel Segmentation

Wide researches have been carried out these years in the domain of retinal vessel segmentation. The algorithms are extensively divided into categories like pattern recognition & classification, matched filtering, vessel tracking, morphological image processing, multi-scale filtering, model based techniques [69]. We studied and extended our research towards supervised pattern recognition techniques. Supervised approach is rule based learning with the help of manually labelled ground truth images also termed as gold standard.

There has been a substantial exploration of ANN for the application to retinal vessel segmentation. Sinthanayothin et al. [70] used PCA for feature extraction accompanied by neural network. The pixel wise feature vector using the Gaussian matched filter and its multiscale derivative was proposed by Niemejer et al. [71]. A k-NN classifier was used to find the probability of pixel being a positive vessel pixel. Staal et al. [72] proposed the technique based on extracting the ridges of the image which run parallel to vessel centrelines and used k-NN classifier for classification. A 2-D Gabor wavelet transform at multiple scales was used in a feature vector by Soares et al. [73]. A Gaussian mixture model (GMM) classifier was used for classification. But the algorithm detected false positives in the presence of pathologies and non-uniform illumination. A feature vector included two orthogonal line detectors in the algorithm given by Ricci and Perfetti [74]. The algorithm needed fewer features and used SVM classifier as a measure to classify the pixels as vessels or not. A 41-D feature vector rich in structural and shape information followed by feature-based AdaBoost classifier (FABC) was proposed by Lupascu [75] for vessel segmentation. You et. al [76] demonstrated a semi supervised approach i.e. training from ground truth as well as weakly labelled data using SVM for vessel segmentation. A multilayer feed forward neural network proposed by Marin et al. [77] is an effective vessel segmentation technique in varied image conditions. A 7-D feature vector employed in the algorithm consists of gray-level and moment invariant-based features. A simplified ensemble approach proposed by Fraz et al. [78] using bagged and boosted decision tree for retinal vessel segmentation obtained good results to be used in retinal image analysis. The another approach using ANN i.e. use of lattice neural network have also been reported by Vega et. al [79] for segmentation of blood vessels. A three layer perceptron ANN having single node at input and output layers was also proposed by Franklin and Rajan [80] for retinal vessel segmentation. The use of GMM classifier and sub-image classification method proposed by Roychowdhary [81] which requires less dependence on training data is an another approach to extract vessels. Zhu et al. [82] used ELM classifier on a discriminative feature vector to segment the retinal vessels.

The use of CNN and ensembled random forest classifier for retinal vessel extraction proposed by Wang et al. [83] surpasses other existing methods. The superpixel generation to reduce the dimensions is one of the prominent features of the method. Fu et al.[84] exploited fully CNN derived from holistically-nested edge detection (HED) problem to generate vessel probability map. The similar kind of CNN approach for extracting retinal vessels is proposed by Hu et al.[85] at multi scales and dilated multi-scale CNN by Jiang et al. [86]. Multiple CNN layers are stacked to create deeper networks which attain improved results. Lisowski et al.[87] proposed a similar deeper CNN architecture for vessel segmentation utilising structured prediction (SP). The architecture makes predictions for all pixels in the patch at a time.

CNN architectures are termed as fully convolutional when dense fully connected layers are removed [88]. Dasgupta and Singh [89] employed fully convolutional architecture using SP for retinal vessel segmentation. Sine-Net proposed by Atli and Gedik [90] used fully convolutional layers network resembling a sine wave and applied series of up sampling and down sampling to get retinal vessel segmented from fundus image. A cross connected CNN (CcNet) architecture which combines some of the layer features in intermediate locations is proposed by Feng et al. [91] to boost feature representation. The transfer learning approach is used by Jiang et al. [92] which utilizes the pre-trained weights from AlexNet presented in [88].

U-Net [93] serves as backbone in various medical image segmentation applications and have brought about a revolutionary change in the performance of semantic segmentation in particular. Retinal vessel segmentation has also been explored in several variants of U-Net. Deformable convolutional block along with U-Net architecture as DU-Net is elaborated in approach proposed by Jin et al. [94]. The receptive field and sampling locations along with the hierarchical features are trained based upon the scale and shape of the vessels. Modified residual block combined with spatial attention block is formed and residual spatial attention network (RSAN) is proposed for retinal vessel extraction by Guo et al. [95]. R2U-Net proposed by Alom et al. [96] utilising the features of U-Net, recurrent CNN and residual network attained better performance on several medical semantic segmentation tasks including retinal vessel extraction. A BCDU-Net [97] utilising the power of U-Net, combined with bidirectional ConvLSTM and dense convolutions obtained state-of-the-art performance in vessel segmentation. Spatial attention U-Net (SAU-Net) along with DropBlock to deal with overfitting issue proposed by Guo et al also extract the retinal vessels in an efficient way. A Dense-UNet with combination of inception module and generative adversarial network is proposed by Guo et al. [98] for retinal vessel segmentation. The skip connections are replaced with dense blocks to fuse features to an added depth.

2.2 Publicly Available Retinal Image Databases

The publicly available retinal image datasets forms a key component in validation of the computer aided algorithms. The training of the classifier and validation of the proposed approaches need the retinal images and reference groundtruth. Thus, several research associations have developed and shared the datasets publicly for further researches to be carried out. The popular datasets with annotations to various retinal normal and abnormal structures are namely ROC [99], DIARETDB [100, 101], DRIVE [71], STARE [102], E-Ophtha [103], Kaggle [104], HEI-MED [105], MESSIDOR [106], Drishti-GS [107], IDRiD [108], REVIEW [109], DRIONS–DB [110], RIGA [111], RIM-ONE [112], CHASE [78], HRF [113], VI-CAVR [114], BioImLab [115], ARIA [116] and INSPIRE-AVR [117]. A detail description of color fundus image datasets used in this thesis is provided below.

ROC: It was a multi-year online competition organized by the University of Iowa. The aim of the challenge was to detect MA, the primary sign of DR. ROC database consists of 50 training images with reference annotations available and 50 test images with no groundtruth available. The ground truths for MA were gathered from four experts.

DIARETDB1: DIARETDB1 is a benchmark database of project ImageRet of the Lappeenranta University of Technology, Finland to evaluate computer aided DR algorithms. Database is a collection of 89 retinal fundus images with the reference ground truth annotated from medical experts for MA, SE, EX and HE. Images were taken using the 50° FOV digital fundus camera with changing imaging settings and resolution of 1500×1152.

DRIVE: Digital Retinal Images for Vessel Extraction is one of the most used databases in which the data is acquired from DR screening program held in the Netherlands. The retinographs were captured using Canon CR-5 non-mydriatic fundus camera having a resolution of 568×584 pixels with 45° FOV. This database consists of 40 images, divided into 20 test and 20 training images. The manually segmented images as groundtruth by experienced ophthalmologists are available for test set along with this database. This database does have groundtruth exclusively for retinal vessels.

E-Ophtha:is a database generated from OPHDIAT Tele-medical network for DR screening to aid the scientific research in DR. This database consists of 463 images with resolution ranging from 1440×960 pixels to 2544×1696 pixels and compressed with JPEG standard. The dataset is divided into two parts as E-Ophtha EX having 82 images and remaining images forms a set of E-Ophtha MA. E-Ophtha EX consist of 47 images with EX and 35 images of healthy retina. Similarly, E-Ophtha MA comprises 148 images containing MA and 233 images of no signs of DR. To the best of our knowledge, E-Ophtha is the first dataset that provided pixel-level annotations for the abnormalities such as EX and MA.

STARE: Structured Analysis of the Retina is another well-known dataset consisting of 397 images, each of size 605×700 collected from Shiley Eye Center at the University of California, San Diego. Topcon TRV-50 fundus camera was used to capture the images at $35°$ FOV. They provide 20 images with the pixel-level hand-drawn ground truth of blood vessels and OD center mark-up for all images. The STARE database consists of 20 images, and there is no division of test and training set in particular.

CHASE: CHASE dataset is prepared with the aim of 'Child Heart And Health Study in England' by Kingston University London. The dataset consist of 28 healthy retina images, each of size 1280×960. Two sets of annotated ground truth are available, out of which first is commonly used.

HRF: High Resolution Fundus is a retina image dataset freely available for research work containing 45 images (15 healthy patients, 15 with DR, 15 with glaucoma), each of high resolution size 3504×2336. The experts working in field of retinal image analysis and ophthalmologists have generated the gold standard ground truth for the dataset.

2.3 Chapter Summary

The chapter presented a review of the literature involved in the contribution to research in the computer aided screening of DR. The thesis includes the algorithms proposed for computer aided screening of retinal vessels and pathologies like MA and EX detection. It sequentially gives a brief to the research and contributions in detecting the MA and EX. Further the review of literature involved in retinal vessel segmentation is discussed. The conventional supervised classification techniques and thereafter the recent ongoing deep learning strategies are elaborated. The publicly available fundus image datasets for retinal screening are enlisted and the datasets used during the thesis are summarized. The next chapter presents our first contribution which is a simple yet effective unsupervised clustering technique for EX detection.

Chapter 3

A K-means clustering approach for exudate detection

3.1 Introduction

Diabetic Retinopathy (DR) is primarily signalized by the occurrence of microa-neurysms, haemorrhages and exudates on the retina. In this contribution, we focus on the DR pathology, that is one of the main indication of an early stage of the disease called intra-retinal lipid exudates, which reflect the breakdown of the blood-retinal barrier. This breakdown of blood-retinal barrier allow access of fluid, rich in lipids and proteins to the parenchyma resulting into exudation and retinal edema [118]. Thus, exudates (EX) are one of the most prevalent lesions at the early stages of DR due to lipid discharge from blood vessels of abnormal retinas. Figure 3.1 shows a fundus image of an unhealthy retina with its main structures and EX.

3.2 Related Work

Several techniques have been proposed for EX detection including the morpholog-ical image processing, supervised and unsupervised way of classification. Walter et

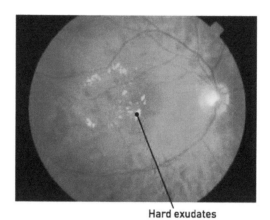

Hard exudates

FIGURE 3.1: Retina Image containing Exudates

al. [29] proposed a method for automated finding of EX in color eye fundus images using mathematical morphology techniques (e.g. morphological reconstruction). Sopharak et al. [30] and [31] described a method very similar to the method as proposed in [29]. However, the limitation of these method is that it produces high false positives. Sopharak et al. [32] also used fuzzy c-means clustering to coarsely detect EX followed by morphological techniques. The inverse surface thresholding approach in [33] finds EX with greater performance indices but fixing a thold is a limitation. The supervised classification method for exudate detection using neural networks have been proposed in [34, 35, 36, 37, 38]. The support vector machine approach in [39], mixture model approach in [40], region growing segmentation algorithms in [41], adaptive fuzzy logic approach in [42] have been also seek to detect EX. They have used different features (colour, illumination, contrast, etc.) assuring the EX detection but at the cost of simplicity. This approach proposed an EX detection technique based on clustering and morphological image processing on retinal images. The technique requires lower computing power and provides acceptable results than other clustering algorithms. The technique works well even for the low contrast images and requires very less computation time.

3.3 Proposed Method

The proposed approach employs an unsupervised clustering technique for detection of EX. The OD might get misdiagnosed as EX area as both have nearly same contrast, so it is required to eliminate the OD area from the retinal images to avoid its intervention in EX detection. Thus, the approach begins with detection of OD and is further extended to extract EX from retinal fundus images.

3.3.1 Optic Disk detection

A bright advent on the retina which is circular in shape is the identification of optic disk (OD). The OD is characterized by the entrance of blood vessels and has high contrast amongst the other circular areas [119]. The hue, saturation and intensity (HSI) space of the original image is used because HSI colour space allows the easy separation of intensity component from the other two colour components. The intensity component of the input image is as shown in Figure 3.3(a). A method similar to the one proposed in [30] is employed for OD detection.

A median filtering operation is applied on an image to attenuate the noise followed by CLAHE for contrast enhancement [120]. Adaptive Histogram Equalization (AHE) is an adaptive method in which several histograms, each analogous to a distinct segment of the image are computed. These are used to redistribute the lightness values of the image. CLAHE is different from ordinary AHE in its contrast limiting. CLAHE is a method that has shown itself to be useful pre-processing tool and in assigning displayed intensity levels in medical images.

OD is characterised by high intensity value and thus contrast stretching assigns the pixels more intensity values. The contrast stretch is often referred to as the dynamic range adjustment. It is a linear transform that maps the lowest gray level $GLmin$ in the image to zero and the highest value $GLmax$ in the image to 255 (for an eight-bit image), with all other gray levels remapped linearly between zero and 255, to produce a high-contrast image that spans the full range of gray levels.

$$Ic_1(x,y) = \left\{ \frac{255}{GLmax - GLmin}[Ip(x,y) - GLmin] \right\} \qquad (3.1)$$

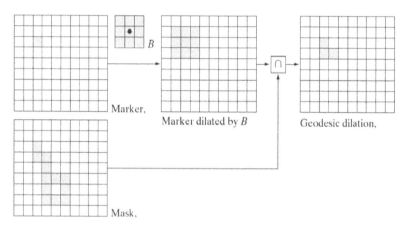

FIGURE 3.2: Morphological reconstruction by Dilation

where Ip is the output image obtained after pre-processing.

The OD brightens due to contrast stretching and its removal from the image becomes easier. The contrast stretched image Ic_1 is as shown in Figure 3.3(b). Morphological reconstruction [121] is a powerful operation in mathematical morphology that inserts the concept of connectivity in images, both for binary and gray scale. Reconstruction is a morphological transformation involving two images and a structuring element (instead of a single image and structuring element). One image, the marker, is the starting point for the transformation. The other image which is used as mask, constrains the transformation. The used structuring element defines connectivity. The image is binarized by using a simple threshold value α_1. Value of $\alpha_1 = 0.9$ gives the acceptable result and the thresholded result I_r is used as a mask. The mask image is inverted before it is superimposed on the original image to remove candidate bright regions. The morphological reconstruction by dilation, R is then applied on the previous superimposed image given as follows,

$$Ic_2 = R_{I_r}(Ic_1) \tag{3.2}$$

To fit the contour of marker image under the mask image, several dilations of marker image Ic_1 under mask image I_r are repeated. The difference of the original image and the reconstructed image is underwent thresholding at grey level α_2

using the following equation.

$$Ic_3 = T_{\alpha_2}(Ip - Ic_2) \tag{3.3}$$

Otsu algorithm is used as a measure for automatic selection of threshold. As a result, high intensities are restored while the rest part is removed, as shown in Figure 3.3(c). Many a times the blood vessels interfere in the circular region of OD. Thus, the reconstructed part does not include the region where vessels were present. Applying a gray scale closing operator ϕ on the resulting image improves the disconnected regions of the optic disk to merge. A flat disc-shaped structuring element with a radius of six S_1 is used.

$$Ic_4 = \phi^{S_1}(Ic_3) \tag{3.4}$$

where S_1 is the morphological structuring element. Normally, the largest circular area can be easily recognized as the OD. However, in some cases there might be huge EX areas in the image which are even larger than the OD. Therefore, the OD region extraction process needs to be made specific to the largest one among the regions whose shapes are circular as it is round in shape [30]. Circularity of the shape of the region is defined by the value of compactness, M, as defined using the following equation:

$$M = \frac{4\pi * A}{P^2} \tag{3.5}$$

where A (area) is the number of pixels in the region and P (perimeter) is the total number of pixels that makes the boundary of each region. The region whose value of compactness is close to one is the most circular. Dilation of the selected result (largest among circular shapes), Ic_5 with a binary dilation operator δ ensures that all pixels in the OD area are covered. In this step, a flat disc-shaped structuring element S_2 with a fixed radius of six is used.

$$OD = \delta^{S_2}(Ic_5) \tag{3.6}$$

The final OD detected after the dilation operation is as shown in Figure 3.3(d).

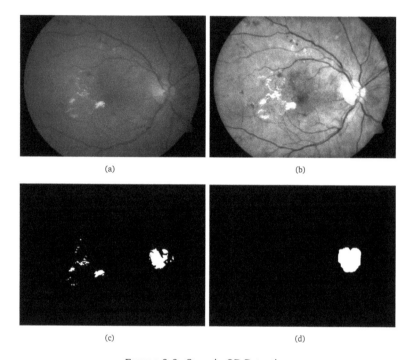

(a)	(b)
(c)	(d)

FIGURE 3.3: Steps in OD Detection

3.3.2 Feature selection

EX can be extracted from retina image on the basis of color, intensity and texture. We attempt to extract these relevant and significant features from the fundus image to differentiate exudate from non-exudate pixels [32]. The green plane of the original image in RGB color space is used as an input in feature selection because lesions have the highest contrast with the background and bulk of the relevant data is contained in this color space. Two features are experientially selected and used as input for K means clustering. The details of feature selection are explained as follows:

1. EX are notable from normal pixels by their gray scale intensity. A median filtering operation is popular in image processing for smoothing and denoising. Here, we use median filtering to distinguish EX from background

pixels. A median filter of window size 25×25 is applied on the green component of RGB image. The resultant image is subtracted from the original gray
scale image. The result of subtraction as shown in Figure 3.4(a) is used as
one of the input feature for K means clustering.

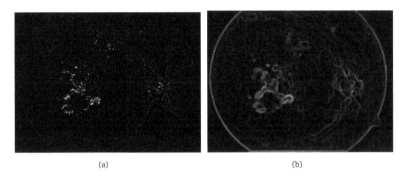

(a)   (b)

FIGURE 3.4: Feature selected for K-means clustering

2. Regions containing EX are characterized by a high grey level and a high
   contrast. Thus, a CLAHE is applied on the green component of input image
   for contrast enhancement. The bright regions and artefacts between dark
   vessels are also characterized by a high local contrast as like EX. So, it is
   required to eliminate the vessels to avoid false positives. A closing operation
   ϕ given as follows serves our purpose:

$$I_{g_1} = \phi^{S_3}(I_g) \tag{3.7}$$

where I_g is the contrast enhanced green component of the image. A structuring element S_3 which is larger than the maximal width of the vessels is
used for closing operation. Further, local variation is calculated for each
pixel in the image. Local variation is chosen as an input parameter because
distribution measurement of the pixel values helps in differentiating exudate
area from the others since it shows the main characterization of the closely
distributed cluster of exudates [29]. Local variation is defined as

$$I_{g_2} = \frac{1}{N-1} \sum_{i \in W(x)} (I_{g_1}(i) - \mu_{I_{g_1}}(x))^2 \tag{3.8}$$

where x is a set of all pixels in a sub-window $W(x)$, N is a number of pixels in $W(x)$, $\mu_{I_{g_1}}(x)$ is mean value of $I_{g_1}(i)$ and $i \in W(x)$. A window size of 9×9 pixels was used in this step. The choice of the size of window is not crucial, but a window size of 9×9 gives satisfactory results. Small isolated EX are often excluded if the window size is chosen too large. The output feature obtained is as shown in Figure 3.4(b).

These two features are used for coarse segmentation of EX using K-means clustering algorithm.

3.3.3 Coarse segmentation of exudate using K means clustering algorithm

K means is a fast and simple unsupervised clustering algorithm which has been used in extraction step to several medical imaging applications. For a brief review of conventional K means algorithm suppose observations are $x_i : i = 1, 2, ..., n$. This clustering algorithm aims to segregate the observations into K groups (clusters) with centroid c_1, c_2,...c_K such that the objective function J is minimized [122].

$$J = \sum_{j=1}^{K} \sum_{i=1}^{n} \left\| x_i^{(j)} - c_j \right\|^2 \tag{3.9}$$

where $\left\| x_i^{(j)} - c_j \right\|^2$ is a chosen distance measure between a data point $x_i^{(j)}$ and the cluster centre c_j, is an indicator of the distance of the n data points from their respective cluster centres.

The input to the K means clustering algorithm is set of features. The algorithm composed is given as follows:

1. Place K points into the space represented by the observation that are being clustered as initial group centroids.

2. Assign each observation to the group that has the closest centroid.

3. Recalculate the positions of the K centroids, when all observations have been assigned

4. Compute the objective function and if the difference between adjacent values of the objective function is less than termination criterion (close to zero or a predefined minimum constant), then stop the iteration; otherwise return to step 2.

The output from the K means clustering is a list of cluster centres and K is a number of desired clusters.

Variance is a measure of how far the observations are spread out. A small variance indicates that the data tends to be very close to the mean and hence to each other, while high variance indicates that the data are dispersed large around the mean and from each other. Experimental results have shown that the cluster with lowest variance extracts most of the EX. The one with lowest value of variance is chosen as an input for fine segmentation of EX using morphological reconstruction. The resulting four clusters are as illustrated in Figure 3.5.

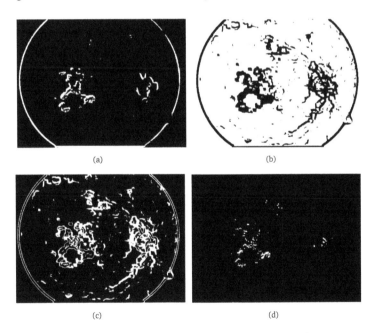

(a)   (b)

(c)   (d)

FIGURE 3.5: Clusters obtained after K-means Clustering

3.3.4 Fine segmentation of exudates by morphological reconstruction

The cluster with minimum variance be I_{mv}. A dilation operator δ of disk shape structuring element S_2 is applied on selected cluster to include all the bordering exudate regions which might have been excluded due to low contrast.

$$I_{dv} = \delta^{S_2}(I_{mv}) \tag{3.10}$$

Morphological reconstruction is carried out on the marker image I_{g_1}. This reconstruction includes the values of pixels next to the candidate regions into the candidate regions by successive geodesic dilation under the mask. As EX are entirely comprised within the candidate region, they are completely removed, whereas non-candidate regions are nearly entirely reconstructed.

The mask image is obtained by setting all the candidate pixels of I_{dv} to zero in the original image. This is done in order to find the contours of EX and to differentiate them from other contrasted regions.

$$I_{dv_1} = \begin{cases} 0 & if \quad I_{dv} \neq 0 \\ I_{g_1} & if \quad I_{dv} = 0 \end{cases} \tag{3.11}$$

Morphological reconstruction by dilation of the resulting image under I_{g_1} is then calculated as follows

$$I_{g_3} = R_{I_{dv_1}}(I_{g_1}) \tag{3.12}$$

The final result is obtained by applying a simple threshold operation to the difference between the original image and the reconstructed image.

$$I_{g_4} = T_{\alpha_2}(I_{g_1} \check{\;} I_{g_3}) \tag{3.13}$$

The OD detected in Section 3.3.1 is subtracted from the above image to get the final result. The stepwise EX detection is illustrated in Figure 3.6.

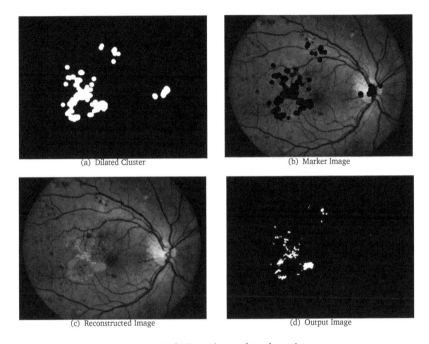

(a) Dilated Cluster   (b) Marker Image

(c) Reconstructed Image   (d) Output Image

FIGURE 3.6: Steps in exudate detection

3.4 Results & Discussion

The section briefs the datasets and performance metrics involved in the evaluation of proposed approach.

3.4.1 Material

The proposed algorithm has been validated on two retinal image datasets DI-ARETDB1 and DRISHTI. 89 images of publicly available DIARETDB1 [101] database were tested on an Intel Core (I5) 2.59 GHz PC using MATLAB R2012a. The performance of our exudate detection technique was evaluated quantitatively by comparing the resulting extractions with ophthalmologist's hand-drawn groundtruth images pixel by pixel. The optic disk detection algorithm was also validated on DIARETDB1 database. OD is perfectly detected in 84 images out of 89. However in some of the images there were some false positives or small parts missing, but the result is still acceptable for our purpose.

We also tested the proposed approach on DRISHTI database, 40 retinal images collected from Drishti Diagnostic Centre, local hospital at Nanded, Maharashtra. But we could not evaluate the performance on this database as annotated groundtruth images are not available.

3.4.2 Evaluation

We evaluated the performance measure of the algorithm at the pixel level using sensitivity and specificity. This pixel based evaluation needs the following four terms. True positive (TP), is the number of correctly detected exudates pixels. False positive (FP) is the number of non-exudate pixels which are incorrectly identified as exudate pixels. False negative (FN), gives the number of exudate pixels that were not detected and true negative (TN) is the number of correctly detected non-exudates pixels [123]. Sensitivity is the measure of pixels correctly classified as lesion by the method.

$$\text{Sensitivity} = \frac{TP}{TP + FN} \tag{3.14}$$

Specificity gives the percentage of correctly classified non-lesion pixels by the method.

$$\text{Specificity} = \frac{TN}{TN + FP} \tag{3.15}$$

Sensitivity and specificity are used to generate receiver operator characteristic (ROC) curve as shown in Figure 3.7. The threshold is varied in the range of 0 to 1. The blue markers in the curve indicate the sensitivity-specificity at various thresholds. An increase in sensitivity is associated with decrease in specificity. There has to be a trade off between two. Thus the system performance is analyzed by calculating the sensitivity and specificity of the algorithm at the optimal threshold [124]. The specificity of the system is less sensitive to change in threshold, varies by a small amount on changing threshold. The sensitivity and specificity

TABLE 3.1: DIARETDB1 results for proposed method for exudate detection

Image	Optic Disk	Sensitivity	Specificity	Image	Optic Disk	Sensitivity	Specificity
1	Yes	0.9963	0.9967	20	Yes	0.6627	0.9966
2	Yes	0.8023	0.9955	21	Yes	0.9842	0.9885
3	Yes	0.9852	0.9977	22	Yes	0.6199	0.9946
4	Yes	0.9889	0.9907	23	Yes	1	0.9932
5	Yes	0.9186	0.9795	24	Yes	0.9926	0.9926
6	Yes	0.9971	0.9962	25	Yes	0.9035	0.9944
7	Yes	0.786	0.9930	27	Yes	0.8158	0.9819
8	Yes	0.6497	0.9877	35	Yes	1	0.9996
9	No	0.8411	0.9838	38	Yes	0.9297	0.9993
10	Yes	0.5469	0.9987	52	Yes	0.8897	0.9962
11	Yes	0.5229	0.9962	53	Yes	0.9811	0.9855
12	Yes	0.9005	0.9995	54	Yes	0.887	0.9894
13	Yes	0.9951	0.9808	66	Yes	1	0.9917
14	Yes	0.9889	0.9946	67	Yes	0.7153	0.9997
15	Yes	0.9521	0.9943	71	Yes	0.6731	0.9995
16	Yes	0.9942	0.9900	84	Yes	0.9902	0.9971
17	Yes	1	0.9888	85	Yes	0.3	0.9998
18	Yes	1	0.9889				
19	Yes	0.8728	0.9864	**Avg**		**0.8834**	**0.9927**

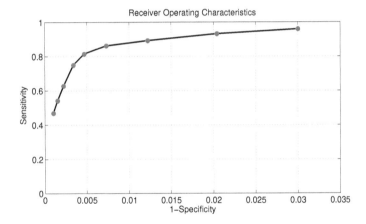

FIGURE 3.7: ROC Curve for the exudate detection on DIARETDB1 database

of the proposed exudate detection algorithm are 88.34% and 99.27% respectively for DIARETDB1 database.

3.4.3 Discussion

The algorithm has shown better results over other existing morphological image processing based methods. The detection of EX by Walter et al. [29] gives the

TABLE 3.2: Comparison of state-of-the-art exudate detection method for DI-ARETDB1 Database

Method	Sensitivity	Specificity
Walter et al. [29]	72.44%	99.67%
Welfer et al. [31]	70.48%	98.84%
Proposed Method	88.34%	99.27%

sensitivity and specificity of 72.44% and 99.67% respectively when tested on DI-ARETDB1 database. The method proposed by Welfer et al. [31] obtained sensitivity and specificity of 70.48% and 98.84% on the same database. The introduction of K means clustering algorithm along with the morphological method helps to find the lesions more effectively.

Thus, we have obtained a relatively greater sensitivity over other existing methods but it can be improved because the low intensity EX pixels are still too subtle to be detected by this algorithm. Our algorithm also has high specificity which showed that the detection of false positives is very less. Figure 3.8 illustrates the obtained results of OD and EX on the random images of DIARETDB1 database. Figure 3.9 illustrates the obtained results of OD and EX on the random images of DRISHTI database.

The automated diagnosis of DR has found to be very useful retinal image analysis. The presented method is not an ultimate application but it can act as a preliminary screening tool or decision support system for ophthalmologists. There are minor misclassification due to the artefacts that are similar to EX and also the artefacts from the noise in the image acquisition process. However, the performance of the algorithm can be improved if the low-contrast EX can also be detected. The inclusion of more specific features to the detection algorithm in the future will assist to increase the sensitivity of the respective system. The incorrect detection of OD in few images also affects the specificity. This suggests the further requisite of improving the method of OD detection.

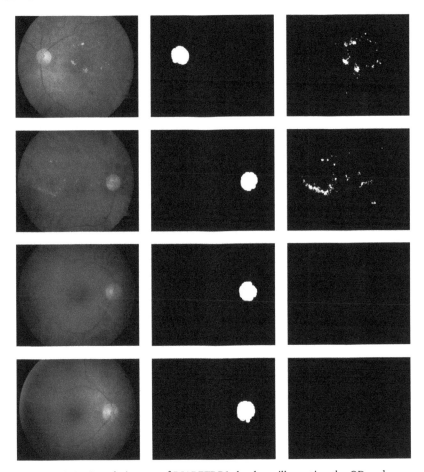

FIGURE 3.8: Sample images of DIARETDB1 database illustrating the OD and exudate detection using proposed method

3.5 Chapter Summary

EX are prominent sign of NPDR which is the vital cause of loss of vision. The chapter presented a method to detect EX from non-mydriatic low-contrast retinal digital images faster and easily. This method detects EX using K-means clustering and morphological image processing on non-dilated pupil and low-contrast retinal images. The OD might get misdiagnosed as EX area due to nearly same contrast

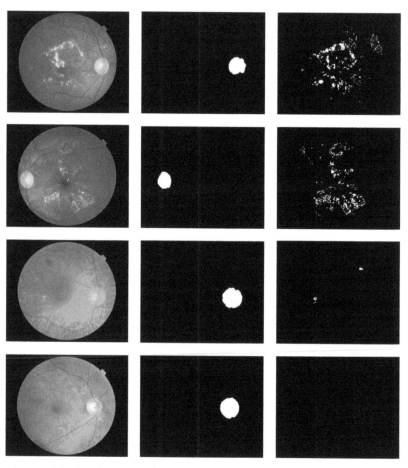

FIGURE 3.9: Sample images of DRISHTI database illustrating the OD and exudate detection using proposed method

as like the EX, so the OD area is detected and eliminated from the retinal images to avoid its intervention in EX detection. The proposed algorithm is validated by comparing the results with expert ophthalmologist's hand-drawn ground truths images available along with DIARETDB1 database. This algorithm is an attempt to help the ophthalmologists in the DR screening process.

Chapter 4

Retinal microaneurysm detection using moment invariant features

4.1 Introduction

In NPDR, the walls of the retinal blood vessels weaken causing leakage of blood and fluid on the retinal surface. Tiny bulges obtrude from the vessel walls and these are microaneurysms (MA) [3]. These bulges are the first clinical appearance of NPDR on retina. Figure 4.1 shows the retinal fundus image with highlighted rectangular region containing MA. MA are red coloured lesions and almost circular in shape. As MA are the first clinical sign of DR, early and accurate detection could obstruct the progress of disease and thus prevent visual impairment. Thus, MA detection plays a significant role in early diagnosis of DR. The lesion detection depends on several imaging conditions and characteristics like illumination, contrast, resolution and other artefacts. Moreover, the varying scale, shape and presence of lesions in the close vicinity of vessels makes the detection of MA more challenging. Computer aided diagnosis (CAD) of DR with the help of advanced image processing techniques is helping eye experts to cope up with these issues.

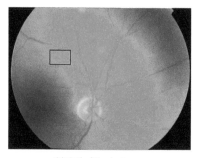

(a) Retinal Fundus Image

(b) Zoom in view of a rectangle containing Microaneurysm

FIGURE 4.1: Retinal Fundus Image containing Microaneurysm

4.2   Related Work

The literature evidences several good researches for the CAD of red lesions. The onset research was based on approaches like mathematical morphology [43], and region growing segmentation [41]. Further supervised and pixel classification methods [44, 46, 52, 53, 55, 58, 60, 66] attained improved performances in MA detection. The other miscellaneous approaches like template matching [50] , sparse representation [49], clutter rejection [51], PCA based unsupervised classification [64], cross section profile analysis [54, 61], differential evolution algorithm [62] were employed for MA detection and achieved competitive results. The number of MA candidates is far less than spurious candidates during the candidate extraction approach, thus class imbalance factor is addressed in several approaches [57, 63, 65]. In recent years, deep learning (DL) is ongoing boom in the area of computer vision and medical image processing. Few papers precisely on the MA detection providing state-of-the-art performance using DL techniques are [17, 18].

4.3   Proposed Method

The approach proposes a novel method for MA detection using moment invariant features and RUSBoost classifier. The potential candidates are extracted from preprocessed image and a set of features comprising of shape, intensity, invariant moments are defined as a representation to each candidate. The class imbalance problem is taken into special consideration and random undersampling boosting classifier is used to improve the performance of classification. Figure 4.2 illustrates the block diagram of the proposed approach.

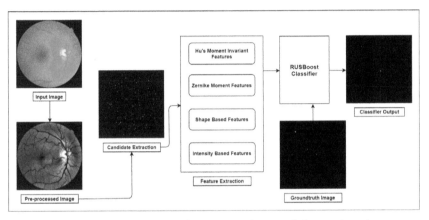

FIGURE 4.2: Block Diagram of the proposed approach for MA detection

4.3.1   Pre-processing

It is important to spot the accurate presence of abnormality in retinal image in spite of poor image characteristics if any. There are several conditions which hamper the retinal image quality during its capture like poor contrast, non-uniform illumination, blurred image, artefacts and others. Pre-processing decreases the effects of noise and retains the characteristics of MA. Thus, pre-processing of retinal images is an essential step during computerised screening of DR.

The green plane of RGB (Red Green Blue) image is used to extract the MA candidates as it holds the highest information and contrast amongst three. A median filter is applied to the green plane of the image (I_g) resulting in an output image (I_{mf}). The median filter (5×5) removes the noise while preserving the edges those analogous to MA. Thereafter, we applied adaptive contrast amplification algorithm to enhance dark structures of image to obtain I_{pp}. The small gaps between bright regions might get incorrectly recognized as MA due to non-uniform illumination.

Thus, a shade correction algorithm is applied to remove bright background variation and thus to repress false positives. A median filter (35×35) applied to I_{pp} gives a background image I_{bg}. Shade corrected image I_{sc} is subtraction of I_{bg} from I_{pp}. The positive pixel value in shade corrected image are the indication of bright regions in I_{pp}. Thus, those bright pixels are replaced by the corresponding pixel value in I_{bg} to obtain the resulting pre-processed image I_p as follows :

$$I_p(i,j) = \begin{cases} I_{bg}(i,j), & \text{if } I_{sc}(i,j) > 0 \\ I_{pp}(i,j), & \text{otherwise} \end{cases}$$

where (i,j) specifies the spatial coordinates of an image.

4.3.2 Candidate Extraction

An effective candidate extraction technique lessens the computation load by detecting the potential MA candidates and decreasing the false positives for analysis in further steps. Thus, it helps in increasing the overall performance of system. Top hat transform along with elongated bounding box rejection criteria is used as candidate extraction approach in this paper. Top hat transform in morphological image processing [121] helps in extracting small elements and details from image. MA are darker than surrounding in retinal image, thus black top hat transform is an operation assists in extracting MA candidates from pre-processed image. The black top hat transform for an image f is given as,

$$T_b(f) = f \bullet b - f$$

where $\bullet$ is the closing operation and b is the structuring element.

Different morphological closing operations are performed on I_{pp} using structuring element of length $l \in L$ at multiple orientation θ ranging from $0°$ to $180°$ with an interval of $15°$ in each orientation. The set of L is fixed such that it is able to find all the possible candidates. The parameter L depends on the size of MA and thus ranges from $\{3, 6, 9, \ldots 60\}$. Experimentally it is found that this set of range extracts all the potential MA candidates. The output of closing operation I_{closed} at different scales is obtained by taking the minimum response over all the considered multiple orientations. The top hat transform score map is then obtained as

$$I_{candidates}^{(l)} = I_{closed}^{(l)} - I_{pp}$$

The score map is then followed by thresholding, where the threshold is calculated so to obtain a maximum of $K = 120$ candidates from the score map. The thresholds t_b are examined from $minimum(I_{candidates}^{(l)})$ to $maximum(I_{candidates}^{(l)})$ with increments of 0.002, so long as the number of connected components in the resulting binary output is smaller than or equal to K. If no lesions are spotted or exceeds K candidates, an experimentally defined lower bound t_l and upper bound t_u are calculate as

$$t_K = \begin{cases} t_l, & \forall t_s : \mathrm{CN}\left(I_{candidates}^{(l)} > t_b\right) < K \\ t_k, & \mathrm{CN}\left(l_{candidates}^{(l)} > t_b\right) \leq K \\ t_u, & \forall t_s : \mathrm{CN}\left(l_{candidates}^{(l)} > t_b\right) > K \end{cases}$$

where CN returns the number of connected components in the score map. A binary output of candidates $B^{(l)}$ at a particular scale l is obtained once the value of threshold t_K is known. The thresholding is repeated at all scales of set L to retain all the possible MA candidates, thus the collective binary map B is obtained as

$$B = \max_{l \in L}(B^{(l)})$$

There are few small candidates in B which are not associated to lesion-based region but add to noise, such connected components less than q_x pixels are removed. q_x should be the minimum number of pixels that a MA lesion contain. An elongated bounding box rejection criteria is also applied to the extracted candidate output image. A bounding box is defined for every candidate of image B. If either length or width of the bounding box exceeds p_x, the candidate is considered to be spurious and rejected as non-MA. This helps in removing the elongated and enlarged candidates which have almost zero chance of being a MA candidate. Experimentally, the value of q_x is found to be 5 pixels and $p_x = 22$. The candidate

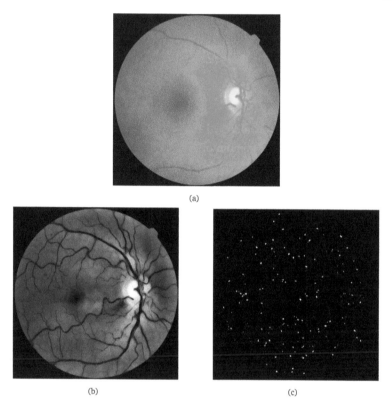

(a)

(b) (c)

FIGURE 4.3: Steps for Candidate Segmentation (a) RGB Image from ROC Dataset (b) Pre-processed Image (c) Candidate Extraction

extraction procedure is illustrated in Algorithm 4.1. Figure 4.3 illustrates the steps in candidate extraction on a randomly chosen image from ROC dataset.

4.3.3 Feature Extraction

Candidate extraction gives all the potential MA regions along with few non-spurious regions. Let the output of candidate extraction stage I_{cand}, a set of N potential candidates be represented as $\{c_1, c_2, c_3, \ldots c_N\}$. Each candidate is represented as a sample feature vector for classification. Extracting accurate descriptors of candidate region is an important step for the success of the ultimate classification

Data: Green Channel of RGB Image I_g,

Result: Image with potential candidates B

Pre-processing:

Median filtering and adaptive contrast amplification I_{pp}

Shade Correction

$$I_{sc} = I_{pp} - I_{bg}$$

for *each pixel (i, j) in I_p* **do**

    if $I_{sc}(i, j) > 0$ **then**

$$I_{bg}(i, j) \leftarrow I_p(i, j)$$

    else

$$I_{pp}(i, j) \leftarrow I_p(i, j)$$

    end

end

Candidate extraction:

for $l = 3;\ l <= 60;\ l = l + 3$ **do**

    for $\theta = 0°;\ l <= 180°;\ l = l + 15°$ **do**

$$I_{closed}^l = \min_\theta(closing(I_p, l, \theta))$$

    end

    Top-Hat Transform:

$$I_{candidates}^{(l)} = I_{closed}^{(l)} - I_{pp}$$

    Thresholding with threshold t_K :

$$t_K = \begin{cases} t_l, & \forall t_s : \mathrm{CN}\left(I_{candidates}^{(l)} > t_b\right) < K \\ t_k, & \mathrm{CN}\left(l_{candidates}^{(l)} > t_b\right) \leq K \\ t_u, & \forall t_s : \mathrm{CN}\left(l_{candidates}^{(l)} > t_b\right) > K \end{cases}$$

$$B^{(l)} = thresholding(I_{candidates}^{(l)}, t_K)$$

end

$$B = \max_{l \in L}(B^{(l)})$$

$n \leftarrow$ number of extracted candidates in B

for $x \leftarrow 0$ **to** n **do**

    if $Area(B(x)) < q_x$ **then**

        $0 \leftarrow B(x)$

    end

end

$B \leftarrow B_1\ m \leftarrow$ number of candidates in B_1

for $x \leftarrow 0$ **to** m **do**

    if $length(BoundingBox(B_1(x))) > p_x \vee width(BoundingBox(B_1(x))) > p_x$ **then**

        $0 \leftarrow B_1(x)$

    end

end

$B_1 \leftarrow I_{cand}$

Algorithm 4.1: Algorithm depicting the steps in candidate extraction for MA detection step. 16 features are extracted as a representation of each candidate to identify true lesions from all the potential candidates. The following subsections present the different features that are found to be useful to describe and classify the red lesions.

4.3.3.1 Moment invariant based features

Hu's moment invariant based features [125] are excellent shape descriptors invariant under size, rotation and scale. Thus, these moments are outstanding descriptors of red lesions and thus included in feature vector. The following paragraph illustrates the calculation of moments for a specified candidate region. Let c_x be the candidate region and 2-D moment of order $(p+q)$ is defined as

$$\mathcal{M}_{pq} = \sum_i \sum_j i^p j^q c_x(i,j) \quad p,q = 0,1,2,\ldots$$

where summations are over the spatial coordinates i and j of the bounding box enclosing the candidate region. $c_x(i,j)$ is the gray level value at coordinate point (i,j)

The corresponding central moment is defined as

$$\upsilon_{pq} = \sum_i \sum_j (i - \bar{i})^p (j - \bar{j})^q c_x(i,j)$$

where,

$$\bar{i} = \frac{\mathcal{M}_{10}}{\mathcal{M}_{00}}, \quad \bar{j} = \frac{\mathcal{M}_{01}}{\mathcal{M}_{00}}$$

The normalized central moment of order (p+q) is defined as

$$\nu_{pq} = \frac{\upsilon_{pq}}{(\upsilon_{00})^\gamma} \quad p,q = 0,1,2,\ldots$$

where,

$$\gamma = \frac{p+q}{2} + 1; \quad (p+q) = 2,3,\ldots$$

	A1	A2	A3	A4	B1	B2	B3	B4
$\phi_1 = |\log(I_1)|$	3.0213	3.1391	3.2218	3.2035	5.3643	5.0817	4.5697	4.3825
$\phi_2 = |\log(I_2)|$	6.0296	6.2781	6.4424	6.3998	10.7286	10.1631	9.1393	8.6641
$\phi_3 = |\log(I_3)|$	11.4535	14.0353	13.1680	14.4001	17.1686	17.1464	16.4729	19.3036
$\phi_4 = |\log(I_4)|$	6.5615	7.6421	7.1446	7.0557	11.7668	11.0031	10.3078	9.9155

TABLE 4.1: Module of the logarithm of invariant moments $\phi_1 - \phi_4$ calculated from the marked circular candidate regions show in Figure 4.4(a).

Hu's seven invariant moments are derived from the above definition of regular moment. Experimentally we found that the following four moments give excellent performance in finding out true red lesions from the potential MA candidates.

$$I_1 = \nu_{20} + \nu_{02}$$

$$I_2 = (\nu_{20} + \nu_{02})^2 + 4\nu_{11}^2$$

$$I_3 = (\nu_{30} - 3\nu_{12})^2 + (3\nu_{21} - \nu_{03})^2$$

$$I_4 = (\nu_{30} + \nu_{12})^2 + (\nu_{21} + \nu_{03})^2$$

The inclusion of remainder three moments increases computation and do not add to classification performance. In addition, the module of logarithm of moment invariants is used in feature vector. The logarithm limits the dynamic range and module prevents the complex values resulting from logarithm of negative moment invariants.

Figure 4.4 shows several candidate regions marked in white on a certain part of image. Few MA and non-MA candidates were chosen from this figure to calculate the moment invariants. Table 4.1 shows the moment values corresponding to each candidate region. There is a noticeable difference in values of true MA lesions and non-MA candidates. The moments have an increase in value if they describe MA candidate and a decrease if vice-versa.

4.3.3.2   Zernike Moments

Zernike moments are the mapping of an image onto a set of complex Zernike polynomials. Since Zernike polynomials are orthogonal to each other, Zernike

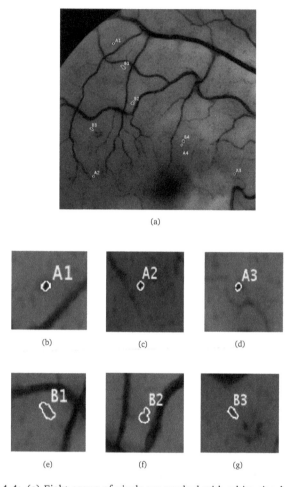

FIGURE 4.4: (a) Eight group of pixels are marked with white circular candidate regions Ak and Bk with k = 1,2,3,4; Ak are microaneurysm pixels whereas Bk are spurious pixels. (b)-(d) are zoomed sub-images of extracted MA pixels, (e)-(g) are zoomed sub-images of extracted spurious objects

moments can represent properties of an image with no redundancy or overlap of information between the moments [126]. Thus, they can be used to extract features that describe the shape of an object. Zernike moments [127] of order n and repetition m for a candidate (region of interest) $c(x, y)$ with size $M \times M$ is

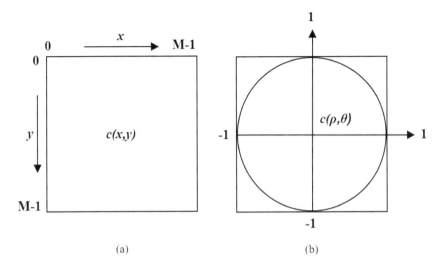

FIGURE 4.5: (a) $M \times M$ size candidate (ROI) with function $c(x,y)$ and (b) function $c(x,y)$ mapped onto unit circle.

defined as

$$Z_{n,m} = \frac{n+1}{\lambda_M} \sum_{x=0}^{M-1} \sum_{y=0}^{M-1} c(x,y) R_{n,m} \left(\rho_{xy}\right) e^{-jm\theta_{xy}} \tag{4.1}$$

where λ_M is a normalization factor which implies the number of pixels inside the unit circle by the mapping transform as shown in Figure 4.5, $R_{n,m}$ is radial polynomial. The mapped distance ρ_{xy} and the phase θ_{xy} at the pixel (x,y) are given as follows:

$$\rho_{xy} = \frac{\sqrt{(2x - M + 1)^2 + (2y - M + 1)^2}}{M}$$

$$\theta_{xy} = \tan^{-1}\left(\frac{M - 1 - 2y}{2x - M + 1}\right)$$

While calculating Zernike moment for a candidate, we make two assumptions. The first is we pad required zeros to either row or column to make candidate of size $M \times M$. The another one is the size of candidate $M \times M$ is always chosen to be even number. The phase value is undefined at center point if size of region of interest is odd, thus selecting an even number solves the problem without any redundancy. The magnitude response of Zernike moments is rotation invariant and the rotation only influences its phase response [127]. Thus, rotation invariant magnitude response of Zernike moments which are the proper shape descriptors are selected as features for our application. The low order Zernike moments are chosen as they are computationally less complex and have low sensitivity to noise. Four moments are selected as features with value of order $n = \{2, 4, 6, 8\}$ and $m = 2$.

4.3.3.3   Shape and Intensity based features

Shape and intensity based features are also added to feature vector to improve the performance of classification. These features portray the overall MA characteristics and assist in classifying true lesions. The description of these local features is as follows:

1. Area ($Area$) : The number of pixels in the candidate region specifies its area.

2. Perimeter ($Peri$) : The number of pixels surrounding the boundary of candidate is defined as its perimeter.

3. Aspect Ratio (AR) : The ratio of length of major axis to the length of minor axis is aspect ratio. The length of major axis and minor axis is nearly same for true MA candidates.

4. Compactness ($Comp$) : The measure of circularity of candidate is defined as its Compactness. Compactness is also near to one for true MA candidates.

$$Comp = \frac{4\pi Area}{Peri^2}$$

5. Solidity (Sol) : The proportion of pixels in convex hull region of candidate i.e. ratio of Area to Convex Area.

6. The measure of intensity at the centroid of the candidate region ($I_{centroid}$).

Notation	Name	Description
$V_1 - V_4$	$\phi_1, \phi_2, \phi_3, \phi_4$	Module of the logarithm of invariant moments
$V_5 - V_8$	$Z_{22}, Z_{42}, Z_{62}, Z_{82}$	Magnitude response of Zernike moments
V_9	$Area$	Area of the candidate region
V_{10}	$Peri$	Perimeter of the candidate region
V_{11}	AR	Ratio of major axis to minor axis
V_{12}	$Comp$	Measure of circularity
V_{13}	Sol	Ratio of Area to Convex Area
V_{14}	$I_{centroid}$	Intensity at centroid of candidate region
V_{15}	I_{mean}	Mean intensity of the candidate region of preprocessed image
V_{16}	I_{min}	Minimum intensity of the candidate region of preprocessed image

TABLE 4.2: Description of features extracted for each candidate region in MA classification

7. The mean intensity of the MA candidate region of the pre-processed image (I_{mean}).

8. The minimum intensity of the MA candidate region of the pre-processed image (I_{min}).

Table 4.2 gives a brief description of all the 16 features extracted for each candidate region to be given as a vector to the classifier.

4.3.4 RUSBoost Classifier

Random Undersampling Boosting (RUSBoost) [128] is a technique effective at classifying imbalanced data. With context to MA classification, we have huge number of non-MA candidates and few MA candidates. Thus, this class imbalance issue is of prime importance to handle, to increase the overall efficiency of the system. Thus, we experimentally found RUSBoost is more suitable and effective classifier to differentiate MA from non-MA candidates and thus address the class imbalance problem. Random undersampling (RUS) randomly removes samples from the majority class till the required class distribution is achieved. The drawback with RUS is the loss of information because of removing samples from training data but is it overcome by its combination with boosting. The simplicity, speed and performance of RUS over other data sampling techniques and the advantages of adaptive boosting algorithm together makes an excellent algorithm for class imbalance classification.

AdaBoosting [129] combine several weak learners into a single ensemble classifier through majority voting. Initially, all the samples are set so as to weigh equally. In each iteration, a model is formed by the base learner and weights are adjusted based on the calculated error. The correctly classified instances are assigned lower weights whereas the weight of misclassified instances is increased. Weak models are trained using weighed instances to rectify the classification of misclassified instances in each iteration. The process is repeated until no further improvement is observed on the training set or a specified number of weak classifiers are formed. In RUSBoost algorithm, a subset is randomly undersampled from the majority class in each iteration of AdaBoost algorithm. The weak learners are then trained using this balanced training set.

The RUSBoost classifier is briefed in Algorithm 4.2. The feature vector $\mathbb{V} = \{V_1, V_2, \ldots V_n\}$ with corresponding labels $\mathbb{Y} = \{y_1, y_2, \ldots y_n\}$ forms a training set. The weight for each instance i in iteration t is denoted as $\mathcal{D}_t(i)$. All weights are set to $\frac{1}{n}$ at start. A class-balanced subset $\mathbb{R}'$ is obtained by randomly undersampling $\mathbb{R}$ set in each iteration. The selected subset $\mathbb{R}'$ and weights $\mathcal{D}'_t$ train the weak learner to minimize error. The weights are updated based on weight update parameter α_t and calculation of pseudo-loss ϵ_t. The updated weights train the next weak learner and this is repeated T times. The final output $H(x)$ which is the probability of the candidate being MA is the weighted combination of T weak learners.

Decision trees are employed as weak learners in RUSBoost algorithm. Decision trees are trained by splitting data from root node to leaves. The required number of splits along with the maximum number of trees at certain shrinkage decides the optimal implementation and performance of decision trees. The addition of trees corrects the residual error resulted due to predictions from the existing trees. But adding too many trees can overfit the training set. Thus, a weighing factor also called as a shrinkage lessens the contribution of each added tree to prevent overfitting. The number of decision trees decide the optimal shrinkage. The selection of parameters is very well experimented and demonstrated in the approach proposed by Dashtbozorg et al. [65]. Thus, we used 100 as maximum number of splits, 1000 as number of weak learners with a weighing factor of 0.5 and obtained significant classification performance of RUSBoost classifier for MA detection.

Data: Set $\mathbb{R}$ of training samples $(V_1, l_1), \ldots, (V_n, l_n)$ where n is number of training samples,
$V_i \in \mathbb{V}$ and $y_i \in \mathbb{Y} = \{-1, +1\}$
Result: $H(x)$
Initialize: $\mathcal{D}_1(i) = \frac{1}{n}$ for all i
for $t = 1$ **to** T **do**
> $\mathbb{R}' \leftarrow$ RUS training set $\mathbb{R}$
> $\mathcal{D}'_t \leftarrow$ weights for the subset $\mathbb{R}'$
> Call $WeakLearn$ with subset $\mathbb{R}'$ and weights $\mathcal{D}'_t$ to train weak classifier h_t
>
> $$h_t = \underset{h_j \in \mathbb{H}}{\operatorname{argmin}} \sum_{1}^{|\mathcal{D}'_t|} \mathcal{D}'_t(i) \left[y_i \neq h_j(V_i)\right]$$
>
> Pseudo-loss calculation for $\mathbb{R}$ and $\mathcal{D}_t$
>
> $$\epsilon_t = \sum_{i=1}^{n} \mathcal{D}_t(i) \left[y_i \neq h_t(V_i)\right]$$
>
> Weight Update Parameter
>
> $$\alpha_t = \frac{1}{2} \ln \frac{1 - \epsilon_t}{\epsilon_t}$$
>
> Update weights and normalization:
>
> $$\mathcal{D}_{t+1}(i) = \mathcal{D}_t(i) \exp\left(-\alpha_t y_i h_t(V_i)\right) / Z_t$$
>
> Normalization Factor
>
> $$Z_t = \sum_{i=1}^{n} \mathcal{D}_{t+1}(i)$$

end
Final Classifier Output

$$H(x) = \sum_{t=1}^{T} \alpha_t h_t(x) / \sum_{j=1}^{T} \alpha_t$$

Algorithm 4.2: Pseudocode for RUSBoost classifier

4.4   Results & Discussion

The section briefs the datasets and performance metrics involved in the validation of proposed approach. The performance of the proposed vessel segmentation method is compared with the existing state-of-the-art approaches based on supervised learning.

4.4.1   Material

We have used three publicly available benchmark datasets to validate our proposed approach: ROC, DIARETDB1 and e-ophtha database.

Retinopathy Online Challenge (ROC) [99] is an online competition which explicitly deals with computer aided MA detection, but new submission is at present not possible. ROC database consists of 50 training images with reference annotations available and 50 test images with no ground truth available. 50 training images are thus used to train and test the proposed approached with k-fold (k=10) cross validation.

DIARETDB1 [101] is a benchmark database collection of 89 retinal fundus images with the reference groundtruth annotated from medical experts. Images were taken using the $50°$ FOV digital fundus camera with changing imaging settings and resolution of 1500×1152.

e-ophtha [103] is a database generated from OPHDIAT Tele-medical network for DR screening to aid the scientific research in DR. It consist of two sub databases, out of which e-ophtha-MA contains images with MA. e-ophtha-MA has 148 images with lesions along with the manually annotated groundtruth by experts.

4.4.2   Evaluation

The proposed approach has been evaluated using repeated 10-fold cross validation procedure. Each dataset is randomly split into 10 equal sized folds. 9 folds are used to train the classifier and the approach is tested using the 10th fold. The cross-validation method has been repeated 10 times, resulting in 10 performance results which are then combined to produce a single estimate.

Free-response operating characteristic (FROC) curve is used to evaluate the performance of proposed MA detection approach. FROC curve is a plot of sensitivities versus the false positives per image (FPI). Sensitivity is the measure of red lesions correctly classified by the classifier. False positives are the non-MA incorrectly classified as red lesions by the classifier. The value of sensitivities at standard FPI values $(1/8, 1/4, 1/2, 1, 2, 4, 8)$ are obtained from the FROC curve for the ease of comparison with the state-of-the-art and the average of all these sensitivities is termed as final FROC score (F_{score}). The partial trapezoidal area under the curve (F_{AUC}) between the above specified range of FPI is also calculated. The comparison table of the proposed approach with the state of the art with reference to F_{score} and F_{AUC} for all the publicly available datasets ROC, DIARETDB1 and e-ophtha is presented in Table 4.3, Table 4.4 and Table 4.5 respectively. The FROC curve for these datasets is depicted in Figure 4.6.

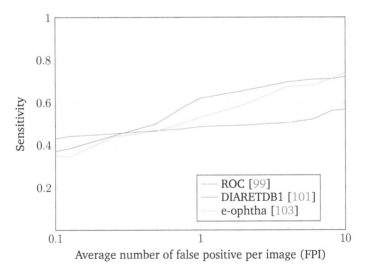

FIGURE 4.6: FROC curve analysis of proposed approach on ROC, DIARETDB1 and e-ophtha dataset
Note: x-axis scale is logarithmic

4.4.3   Discussion

The variability in spatial resolution and presence of artefacts makes the detection of MA more challenging in ROC dataset. The proposed method however, overcomes these problems and attains an overall average (F_{score}) of 0.496, which outperforms the existing MA detection methods. Table 4.3 shows the comparison of sensitivity v/s predefined FPI (false positive per image) of the proposed approach with the state-of-the-art methods. The clinical expert provides 1.08 FPI as an indication of "clinically acceptable" and suggests that it brings out the higher performance of the system during the CAD in clinical environments. Though few approaches as like proposed by Antal and Hazdu [53], Wang et al. [61], Dai et al [57], Derwin et al. [68] report higher sensitivities at 2 and above FPI, our proposed approach excels at $\{1/8, 1/4, 1/2, 1\}$ FPI values.

The proposed method also outperforms on DIARETDB1 dataset, even in presence of artefacts and dark spots in most of the images of dataset. Table 4.4 illustrates the comparison of the proposed approach with existing ones on DIARETDB1 dataset. The method attains F_{score} of 0.571 and the area under curve (F_{AUC}) of 0.655, which is significantly better compared to state-of-the-art methods. The approach performs satisfactory on e-ophtha database with F_{score} of 0.537. The method proposed by Chudzik et al. [18] excels in performance on e-ophtha dataset but it attains lower values on ROC and DIARETDB1 datasets. The comparison with the literature depicts that the proposed approach performs competitive with respect to all the datasets used for validation. We have employed RUSBoost classifier in the proposed method with an aim to deal with the majority class imbalance perspective. Thus, the comparison of the proposed approach with the methods employing class-imbalance approaches for MA detection is illustrated using FROC curve on respective datasets as shown in Figure 4.7, Figure 4.8 and Figure 4.9. Though the approach proposed by Dai et al. [57] records higher sensitivity values at higher FPI in ROC dataset, the proposed method has overall higher F_{score}. Moreover, the proposed approach has highest sensitivity at 1.08 FPI when compared to the other ones. Table 4.6 illustrates randomly selected RGB fundus images from the datasets along with its groundtruth and final output achieved by the proposed algorithm. It is apparent from the Table 4.6 that the proposed method attains a strong output when compared with groundtruth results.

The complete automated MA detection approach has been developed in MATLAB 2017b environment using an Intel Core i5-7300HQ CPU at 2.50 GHz. The average time required for computation per image is about 50 seconds.

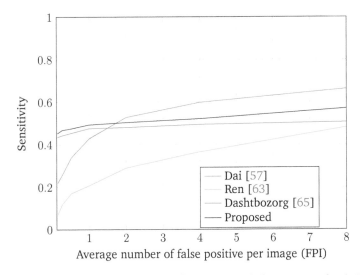

FIGURE 4.7: FROC curve analysis for different class-imbalance approaches in MA detection on ROC dataset

4.5   Chapter Summary

As MA are first clinical sign of DR, early and precise detection of MAs could hinder the development of the disease. The chapter investigated a novel method for the accurate detection of MA in retinal fundus image. A supervised classification approach is presented by extracting the moment invariant features along with the intensity and shape based features. The candidates extracted from pre-processed image consist of MA as well as spurious candidates. The small number of true MA candidates in comparison to non-MA candidates makes it a class imbalance problem, thus RUSBoost classifier is used which deal with the class imbalance issue. The proposed approach is validated on three publicly available datasets viz. ROC, DIARETDB1 and e-ophtha. The method outperforms the existing state-of the-art methods and evidences its ability for use in automated screening of DR.

Method	Sensitivity against FPI							F_{score}	F_{AUC}
	1/8	1/4	1/2	1	2	4	8		
Proposed Method	0.453	0.468	0.475	0.493	0.504	0.521	0.560	**0.496**	0.513
Derwin et al. [68]	0.267	0.331	0.420	0.486	0.535	0.634	0.698	0.481	**0.587**
Dashtbozorg et al. [65]	0.435	0.443	0.454	0.476	0.481	0.495	0.506	0.471	0.484
Wang et al. [61]	0.273	0.379	0.398	0.481	0.545	0.576	0.598	0.464	0.543
Antal and Hazdu [53]	0.173	0.275	0.380	0.444	0.526	0.599	0.643	0.434	0.551
Dai et al. [57]	0.219	0.257	0.338	0.429	0.528	0.598	0.662	0.433	0.553
Lazar and Hazdu [54]	0.251	0.312	0.350	0.417	0.472	0.542	0.615	0.423	0.510
Niemeijer et al. [44]	0.243	0.297	0.336	0.397	0.454	0.498	0.542	0.395	0.469
Quellec et al. [50]	0.166	0.230	0.318	0.385	0.434	0.534	0.598	0.381	0.489
Zhang et al. [49]	0.175	0.242	0.297	0.370	0.437	0.493	0.569	0.369	0.465
Adal et al. [56]	0.204	0.255	0.297	0.364	0.417	0.478	0.532	0.364	0.446
Zhang et al. [48]	0.198	0.265	0.315	0.356	0.394	0.466	0.501	0.357	0.430
Sanchez et al. [47]	0.190	0.216	0.254	0.300	0.364	0.411	0.519	0.322	0.399
Fujita Lab [46]	0.181	0.224	0.259	0.289	0.347	0.402	0.466	0.310	0.378
Ram et al. [51]	0.041	0.160	0.192	0.242	0.321	0.397	0.493	0.264	0.368
Kar and Maity [62]	0.061	0.098	0.15	0.222	0.289	0.354	0.382	0.222	0.313
Wu et al. [60]	0.037	0.056	0.103	0.206	0.295	0.339	0.376	0.202	0.302
Chudzik et al. [18]	0.039	0.067	0.141	0.174	0.243	0.306	0.385	0.193	0.281

TABLE 4.3: Comparison of state-of-the-art MA detection methods at predefined FPI for ROC dataset

Method	Sensitivity against FPI							F_{score}	F_{AUC}
	1/8	1/4	1/2	1	2	4	8		
Proposed Method	0.383	0.443	0.5	0.61	0.655	0.695	0.71	**0.571**	**0.655**
Dashtbozorg et al. [65]	0.507	0.517	0.519	0.542	0.555	0.574	0.617	0.547	0.565
Chudzik et al. [18]	0.187	0.246	0.288	0.365	0.449	0.570	0.641	0.392	0.513
Seoud et al. [58]	0.140	0.175	0.250	0.323	0.440	0.546	0.642	0.354	0.495
Dai et al. [57]	0.035	0.058	0.112	0.254	0.427	0.607	0.755	0.321	0.527
Adal et al. [56]	0.024	0.033	0.045	0.103	0.204	0.305	0.571	0.184	0.308
Antal and Hazdu [53]	0.001	0.003	0.009	0.020	0.059	0.140	0.257	0.070	0.130

TABLE 4.4: Comparison of state-of-the-art MA detection methods at predefined FPI for DIARETDB1 dataset

Method	Sensitivity against FPI							F_{score}	F_{AUC}
	1/8	1/4	1/2	1	2	4	8		
Proposed Method	0.352	0.438	0.465	0.53	0.588	0.675	0.71	0.537	0.625
Chudzik et al. [18]	0.185	0.313	0.465	0.604	0.716	0.801	0.849	**0.562**	**0.734**
Dashtbozorg et al. [65]	0.358	0.417	0.471	0.522	0.558	0.605	0.638	0.510	0.575
Wu et al. [60]	0.063	0.117	0.172	0.245	0.323	0.417	0.573	0.273	0.386

TABLE 4.5: Comparison of state-of-the-art MA detection methods at predefined FPI for e-ophtha dataset

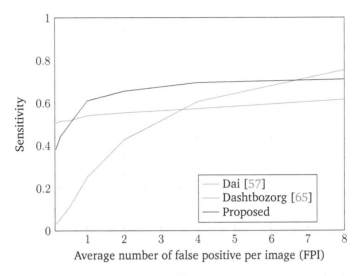

FIGURE 4.8: FROC curve analysis for different class-imbalance approaches in MA detection on DIARETDB1 dataset

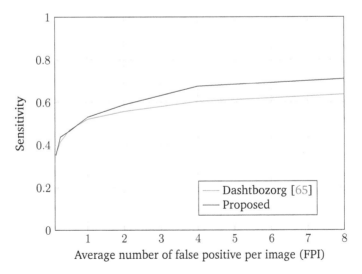

FIGURE 4.9: FROC curve analysis for different class-imbalance approaches in MA detection on e-ophtha dataset

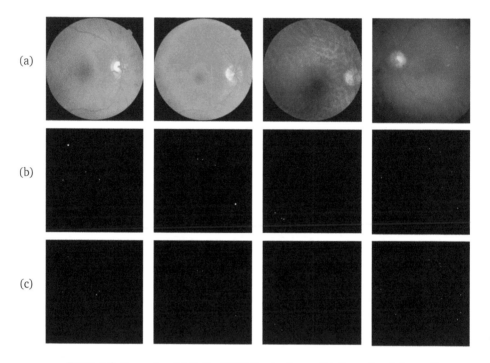

TABLE 4.6: Row-wise: (a) Retinal RGB Fundus Image (b) Groundtruth Image for the RGB image of respective column (c) Final Output Image after classification stage.

Chapter 5

Retinal vessel segmentation using EFMMNN classifier

5.1 Introduction

DR causes damage to blood vessels of the retina. The damage to blood-retinal barrier causes the abruption of vessels and leakage of blood onto the retinal surface. The early indicators of DR at this stage are microaneurysms (MA) and exudates (EX). The advance stages of the disease include the proliferation of new blood vessels and also may lead to retinal detachment. Thus, retinal vessel segmentation is often a pre-requisite during ever stage of DR screening as well as in image registration. The retinal vessel extraction is a challenging task due to uneven intensity distribution, complex structure of thin and tiny vessels, image distortion & artefacts included during its capture and several other imaging conditions. Accurate segmentation of vessels are of considerable clinical significance due to its potential predictive role in determining the development of future risks in DR. Wide researches have been carried out during recent years in the domain of retinal vessel segmentation.

5.2   Related Work

There has been a substantial exploration of artificial neural network for the application to retinal vessel segmentation. Sinthanayothin et al. [70] used PCA for feature extraction accompanied by neural network. The pixel wise feature vector using the Gaussian matched filter and its multiscale derivative followed by k-NN classifier was proposed by Niemejer et al. [71]. Staal et al. [72] proposed the technique based on extracting the ridges of the image which run parallel to vessel centrelines and used k-NN classifier for classification. A 2-D Gabor wavelet transform at multiple scales was used in a feature vector by Soares et al. [73]. A feature vector included two orthogonal line detectors and SVM for classification in the algorithm given by Ricci and Perfetti [74]. A 41-D feature vector rich in structural and shape information followed by feature-based AdaBoost classifier (FABC) was proposed by Lupascu [75] for vessel segmentation. You et. al [76] demonstrated a semi supervised approach i.e. training from ground truth as well as weakly labelled data using SVM for vessel segmentation. Moment invariant-based features and multilayer feed forward neural network employed by Marin et al. [77] was a effective vessel segmentation technique in varied image conditions. A simplified ensemble approach proposed by Fraz et al. [78] using bagged and boosted decision tree for retinal vessel segmentation obtained good results. The another approach using ANN i.e. use of Lattice Neural Network have also been reported by Vega et. al [79] for segmentation of blood vessels. A three layer perceptron ANN having single node at input and output layers was also proposed by Franklin and Rajan [80] for retinal vessel segmentation. The use of CNN and ensembled random forest classifier for retinal vessel extraction proposed by Wang et al. [83] surpasses other existing methods. The use of GMM classifier and sub-image classification method proposed by Roychowdhary [81] which requires less dependence on training data is an another approach to extract vessels. Zhu et al. [82] used ELM classifier on a discriminative feature vector to segment the retinal vessels.

Despite the several ongoing research in several domains, the several challenges involved in vessel segmentation still provides room for improved performance. Thus, a supervised classification approach is elaborated in this work for retinal vessel segmentation based on enhanced fuzzy min-max neural network (EFMMNN)

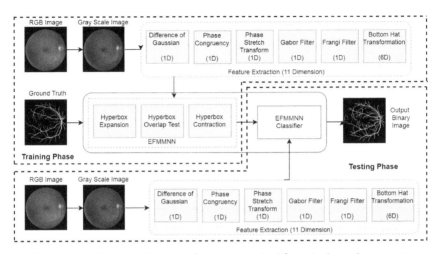

FIGURE 5.1: Schematic Diagram of proposed method for retinal vessel segmentation

[130]. A 11-D feature vector which include spatial as well as frequency domain information, is an input feature to the neural network, trains the network by forming hyperboxes of the distinct classes. In testing phase, the input pattern is fed to the hyperbox layer which makes a decision of a class to which it belongs. This is a two class problem, thus the output is binary deciding whether the pixel belongs to a vessel or not. The publicly available databases along with groundtruth of retina images viz. DRIVE and STARE datasets are used for validation of the proposed approach.

5.3 Proposed Method

The schematic work flow of the proposed method is summarized in Figure 5.1. Though a conventional supervised learning approach is opted, the FMMNN based hyperbox classifier is essence of the algorithm. The following section elaborates the proposed method, beginning with the feature extraction as no pre-processing is involved.

5.3.1 Feature Extraction

Features are the representation of the structure which is to be classified. Selecting appropriate input features is an significant requirement for accurate classification, thus focussed experimental investigations along with the theoretical concept have been taken into consideration while selecting the particular feature. Retinal vessels are analogous to edges and lines in the retinal image. Thus, the spatial and frequency features which highlight high frequency components are chosen as the required features for vessel segmentation.

The RGB fundus image is converted to gray scale and is used without any preprocessing. The gray scale component signifies the intensity of image, thus helpful in edge detection and also reduces the computational complexity over color images. An 11-D feature vector comprising of features like Difference of Gaussian (DoG), phase stretch transform (PST), phase congruency, Gabor filter, Frangi filter, black top-hat transformation is extracted for every pixel of gray scale component of fundus image. This section presents an overview of each feature as follows:

5.3.1.1 Difference of Gaussian

Difference of Gaussian is the subtraction of one smoothed image from another less smoothed version of the same image. The smoothed images are the result of convolution of gray scale images with Gaussian kernels having distinct standard deviations. The spatial information between the range of frequencies that are retained in two smoothed images, is preserved as a result of subtraction. Thus, DoG passes the frequency components analogous to the edges present in the image. Mathematically DoG filter is expressed as,

$$h(x,y) = g_{\sigma_1}(x,y) - g_{\sigma_2}(x,y) \tag{5.1}$$

where $g_{\sigma_1}(x,y)$ and $g_{\sigma_2}(x,y)$ are Gaussian kernels with distinct standard deviation σ_1 and σ_2 expressed as,

$$g_\sigma(x,y) = \frac{1}{2\pi\sigma^2}\exp(-\frac{x^2+y^2}{2\sigma^2}) \tag{5.2}$$

The image output of DoG using convolution is expressed as

$$I_d(g) = I_g * h \qquad (5.3)$$

where I_g is gray scale image. The output of DoG is as shown in Figure 5.2(b).

5.3.1.2 Phase Stretch Transform

Image features like step edges and lines both give rise to pixel points where the Fourier components of the fundus image are maximally in phase. This sharp transitions contain high frequency components and thus PST emphasizes edge information. PST [131] is formulated as

$$I_{PST}[x, y] = \measuredangle \langle IFFT2\{K_p[u, v].L[u, v].FFT2\{I_g[x, y]\}\}\rangle \qquad (5.4)$$

where $I_{PST}[x, y]$ is the output image, $L(u, v)$ is the frequency response of kernel, $\measuredangle$ is the angle operator, $FFT2$ is 2-D Fast Fourier Transform, $IFFT2$ is 2-D Inverse Fast Fourier Transform.

A particular phase kernel is selected for PST operation such that the kernel phase derivative is a linear function with respect to frequency variable. An inverse tangent function that forms a kind of phase kernel is given as

$$K_p[u, v] = \exp^{j.\varphi[u,v]} \qquad (5.5)$$

The kernel phase for the following PST is given as

$$\varphi[u, v] = S.\frac{W.z.tan^{-1}(W.z) - (1/2).ln(1 + (W.z)^2)}{W.z_{max}.tan^{-1}(W.z_{max}) - (1/2).ln(1 + (W.z_{max})^2)} \qquad (5.6)$$

where $z = \sqrt{u^2 + v^2}$. The accurate extraction of high frequency components i.e. edge information requires the precise selection of Strength (S) and Warp (W) of the phase kernel. The bandwidth of the localization kernel also needs to be designed to extract the needed edges. Figure 5.2(c) shows the output feature image of phase stretch transform.

5.3.1.3 Phase Congruency

Congruency of phase at ány orientation infers a clearly perceived feature. It is a dimensionless measure and is invariant to changes in illumination. Phase congruency describes the image in the frequency domain. The efficient measure of phase congruency proposed by Kovesi [132] is defined as

$$I_{PC}(x,y) = \frac{\Sigma_\theta \Sigma_k w_\theta(x,y) \lfloor A_{k,\theta} \Delta\Phi_{k,\theta}(x,y) - T_\theta \rfloor}{\Sigma_\theta \Sigma_k A_{k,\theta}(x,y) + \epsilon} \tag{5.7}$$

where θ is the orientation that spans the range $[0 - \pi]$ with the interval of $\pi/6$. T_θ is the noise response. $\lfloor A_{k,\theta} \Delta\Phi_{k,\theta}(x,y) - T_\theta \rfloor$ denotes that the residing quantity is zero if its value is negative and remains the same otherwise. $\Delta\Phi(x,y)$ is a phase deviation function given as

$$\Delta\Phi(x,y) = cos(\phi_k(x,y) - \phi(x,y)) - |sin(\phi_k(x,y) - \phi(x,y))| \tag{5.8}$$

The weighing function is constructed as a result of applying a sigmoid function to the spread of filter response.

$$w(x,y) = \frac{1}{1 + e^{\gamma_{PC}(c - s(x,y))}} \tag{5.9}$$

where c is the cut-off value and γ_{PC} is a gain factor that controls the cut-off sensitivity. w is a weighing factor that enhances phase congruency at locations where filter response is spread over wide range of frequencies. This prevents spotting of false positives in the region of narrow frequency spread. This spread is given as

$$s(x,y) = \frac{1}{K} \frac{\Sigma_k A_k(x,y)}{A_{max}(x,y) + \epsilon} \tag{5.10}$$

where K is total number of scales and A_{max} is filter amplitude having maximum response. Phase Congruency feature output is as depicted in Figure 5.2(d).

5.3.1.4 Frangi filter

A vesselness measure defined by Frangi [133] based on the eigenvalues of the Hessian matrix is of great help in detecting vessel-like structures. The concept is illustrated in detail in [133].

The signs and ratios of the eigenvalues marks an indication of a local structure. Let λ_1 and λ_2 are the eigenvalues of Hessian Matrix H and $|\lambda_2| \geq |\lambda_1|$. The larger eigenvalue, λ_2 corresponds to the maximum principal curvature at the location (x, y).

A vesselness measure defined by Frangi to feature vessel-like structures is given as

$$V_F = \begin{cases} \exp\left(-\frac{R_\beta^2}{2\beta^2}\right)[1 - \exp\left(-\frac{S_F^2}{2\gamma_f^2}\right)], & \text{if} \lambda_1, \lambda_2 < 0 \\ 0, & \text{otherwise} \end{cases} \tag{5.11}$$

where $R_\beta = \frac{\lambda_1}{\lambda_2}$ and $S_F = \sqrt{\lambda_1^2 + \lambda_2^2}$ is the Frobenius norm of the Hessian matrix and γ_f equals one-half of the maximum of all of the Frobenius norms computed for the whole image. Figure 5.2(e) is the output of Frangi filtering.

5.3.1.5 Gabor filter

Gabor filter has been extensively used for edge detection as it gives high values for high frequency components which are analogous to edges. The center symmetric Gabor filter feature is expressed as:

$$G_v(\mathbf{x}, \Lambda, \theta, \sigma_x, \sigma_y) = \exp\left(\frac{x'^2}{2\sigma_x^2} + \frac{y'^2}{2\sigma_y^2}\right) * cos(2\pi x/\Lambda) \tag{5.12}$$

$$x' = xcos(\theta) + ysin(\theta) \tag{5.13}$$

$$y' = -xsin(\theta) + ycos(\theta) \tag{5.14}$$

where $\mathbf{x} = (x, y)$ is a 2-D point, Λ represents the wavelength of the sinusoidal factor, θ represents the orientation.

σ_x is the sigma of the Gaussian envelope in x direction and hence controls the bandwidth of filter, σ_y controls the sigma across the filter and hence orientation selectivity. For each considered scale value $(\Lambda, \sigma_x, \sigma_y)$, the maximum response over all orientations is found at every pixel, denoted as,

$$M(\mathbf{x}, \Lambda, \sigma_x, \sigma_y) = \arg\max_{\theta \in \oplus} \| G_v(\mathbf{x}, \Lambda, \theta, \sigma_x, \sigma_y) \| \tag{5.15}$$

where $\oplus = \{k\pi/15, k = 0, 1, 2....11\}$. The Gabor filter output i.e. maximum response is as shown in Figure 5.2(f).

5.3.1.6 Black Top-Hat Transformation

The subtraction of image with its closing by some structuring element results in black top-hat transform [121]. The black top-hat transform is used for extracting dark objects on a light background and also corrects non uniform illumination. In a retinal image, vessel pixels are darker than the background. Hence, it is a suitable feature to extract vessels. The black top-hat transform of the gray scale image I_g is given by

$$G_n^\theta = I_g \cdot S_n^\theta - I_g \tag{5.16}$$

where S is a linear structuring element. There is a vivid range of vessel width varying from 2-20 pixels or more depending on the resolution of images. Hence we use multi-scale structuring element that span the entire range and in the step of 4. In every scale, the linear structuring element of the transform spans over all range of orientation $\theta, \theta \in R, R = (m\pi/6, m = 0, 1, ...5)$. Then the maximum value over entire range is selected as the response for individual scale given as

$$G_n = \max_{\theta \in R}(G_n^\theta) \tag{5.17}$$

The output of black top-hat transformation across the six scales is as shown in Figure 5.3.

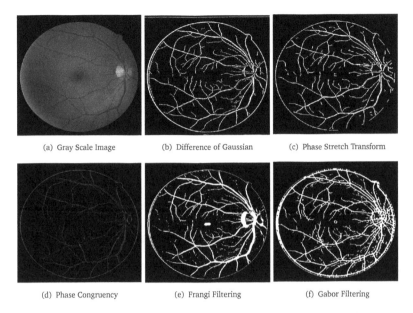

FIGURE 5.2: (a) Gray Scale Image; Illustration of extracted features for vessel segmentation: (b) Difference of Gaussian, (c) Phase Stretch Transform, (d) Phase Congruency, (e) Frangi filtering, (f) Gabor filtering

5.4   Classification

5.4.1   Enhanced Fuzzy Min-Max Neural Network

There have been a wide research on developing intelligent neural networks in combination with fuzzy systems. The fuzzy min max (FMM) networks in combination with artificial neural networks (ANN) overcome the limitations faced by the ANN. The online learning ability and shorter training time makes fuzzy min-max neural network more beneficial for pattern classification [134]. The 'hyperbox' concept in FMM avoids the retraining issue faced by ANN. The online learning ability of FMM helps in solving stability plasticity dilemma. The non-linear separability amongst classes is also a key feature in FMM networks. Thus, a less complexity of FMM implemented in combination with ANN, assists in an easy training and evaluation of vessel extraction from retinal images. The EFMMNN addresses classification

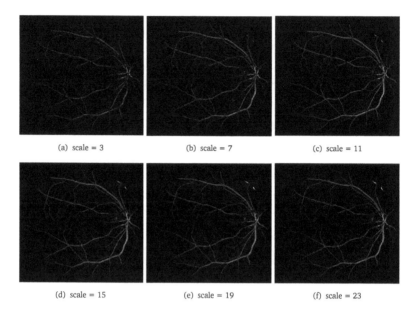

(a) scale = 3   (b) scale = 7   (c) scale = 11

(d) scale = 15   (e) scale = 19   (f) scale = 23

FIGURE 5.3: Features extracted using black top-hat transformation at different scales

problem in a competent way as compared to other existing neural network classifiers stated in the literature. The fuzzy min-max pattern classification is primarily a three step process:

1. Hyperbox Expansion

2. Hyperbox Overlap Test

3. Hyperbox Contraction

The basis of FMM learning is formation of hyperbox based on the given data sample [135]. A training data set comprise of feature vector (as input pattern) and target classes together as ordered pair, F_h where $h = 1, 2, ...H$, H is total no. of data samples. Each hyperbox fuzzy set B_j is represented by a minimum and maximum point in an n-dimensional space within a unit hypercube given as

$$B_j = (F_h, p_j, q_j, f(F_h, p_j, q_j)) \; \forall \; F_h \in I^n \qquad (5.18)$$

where, $F_h = f_{h1}, f_{h2}, ...f_{hn}$ is a feature vector, $p_j = (p_{j1}, p_{j2}, ...p_{jn})$ and $q_j = (q_{j1}, q_{j2}, ...q_{jn})$ are the minimum and maximum points of B_j, respectively.

An input pattern is included in hyperbox when the pattern has full class membership for the given hyperbox. An expansion co-efficient Θ is defined which regulates the size of hyperbox. The membership function is calculated for each new incoming input pattern, to decide its inclusion in the respective hyperbox. The membership function is given as,

$$B_j(F_h) = \frac{1}{2n}\Sigma_{i=1}^n[max(0, 1 - max(0, \gamma min(1, f_{hi} - q_{ji})))+$$
$$max(0, 1 - max(0, \gamma min(1, p_{ji} - f_{hi}))] \qquad (5.19)$$

where γ is the sensitivity regulating factor of membership and inversely proportional to distance between F_h and B_j.

The FMM neural network is a three layered structure as shown in Figure 5.4. F_A is the input layer with no. of nodes equal to length of feature vector. The middle hyperbox layer F_B symbolizes implemented fuzzy rules. Each node in this layer is a hyperbox fuzzy set formed during the FMM training phase. The minimum and maximum points which form the hyperbox are connections between layer 1 and 2 stored in matrices P and Q, respectively. The transfer function of the middle layer is membership function. F_C is the output layer with two nodes; each node corresponds to a class. The matrix U formed as a result of connections between layer 2 and 3 is defined as,

$$u_{jk} = \begin{cases} 1, & \text{if } b_j \in O_k \\ 0, & \text{otherwise} \end{cases} \qquad (5.20)$$

were b_j is j^{th} node of F_B and O_k is k^{th} node of F_C.

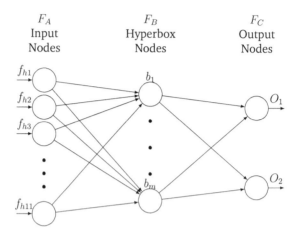

FIGURE 5.4: EFMMNN for the proposed method

5.4.1.1 Hyperbox Expansion

Hyperbox B_j is expanded in order to include the feature input in its corresponding hyperbox class, but only if hyperbox size do not go beyond the expansion co-efficient Θ. So, the following condition needs to be met to expand hyperbox B_j for inclusion of new input pattern in it,

$$Max_n(Q_{ji}, f_{hi}) - Min_n(P_{ji}, f_{hi}) \leq \Theta \tag{5.21}$$

whereby $0 \leq \Theta \leq 1$. Q_{ji} and P_{ji} are the maximum and minimum points of hyperbox B_j along i^{th} dimension. Every dimension of hyperbox B_j is checked individually and the expansion is done provided that all hyperbox dimensions do not exceed expansion co-efficient Θ. If the condition in equation is not met, a new hyperbox is formed to include the pattern.

5.4.1.2 Hyperbox Overlap Test

This above expansion process might result in an undesirable overlap amongst hyperboxes. Thus, an overlap test is needed to check the overlap between two hyperboxes of different classes. The following nine cases illustrates the overlap test for the ith dimension.

- Case 1

$$P_{ji} < P_{ki} < Q_{ji} < Q_{ki}$$
$$\delta^{new} = min(Q_{ji} - P_{ki}, \delta_{old}) \qquad (5.22)$$

- Case 2

$$P_{ki} < P_{ji} < Q_{ki} < Q_{ji}$$
$$\delta^{new} = min(Q_{ki} - P_{ji}, \delta_{old}) \qquad (5.23)$$

- Case 3

$$P_{ji} = P_{ki} < Q_{ji} < Q_{ki}$$
$$\delta^{new} = min(min(Q_{ji} - P_{ki}, Q_{ki} - P_{ji}), \delta_{old}) \qquad (5.24)$$

- Case 4

$$P_{ji} < P_{ki} < Q_{ji} = Q_{ki}$$
$$\delta^{new} = min(min(Q_{ji} - P_{ki}, Q_{ki} - P_{ji}), \delta_{old}) \qquad (5.25)$$

- Case 5

$$P_{ki} = P_{ji} < Q_{ki} < Q_{ji}$$
$$\delta^{new} = min(min(Q_{ji} - P_{ki}, Q_{ki} - P_{ji}), \delta_{old}) \qquad (5.26)$$

- Case 6

$$P_{ki} < P_{ji} < Q_{ki} = Q_{ji}$$
$$\delta^{new} = min(min(Q_{ji} - P_{ki}, Q_{ki} - P_{ji}), \delta_{old}) \qquad (5.27)$$

- Case 7

$$P_{ji} < P_{ki} \leq Q_{ji} < Q_{ki}$$
$$\delta^{new} = min(min(Q_{ji} - P_{ki}, Q_{ki} - P_{ji}), \delta_{old}) \tag{5.28}$$

- Case 8

$$P_{ki} < P_{ji} \leq Q_{ki} < Q_{ji}$$
$$\delta^{new} = min(min(Q_{ji} - P_{ki}, Q_{ki} - P_{ji}), \delta_{old}) \tag{5.29}$$

- Case 9

$$P_{ki} = P_{ji} < Q_{ki} = Q_{ji}$$
$$\delta^{new} = min(Q_{ki} - P_{ji}, \delta_{old}) \tag{5.30}$$

δ^{new} is the minimum overlap value for the respective case. If an overlap is found between two hyperboxes of different classes, a hyperbox contraction is required to prevent the misclassification and remove the overlap between two.

5.4.1.3   Hyperbox Contraction

When there is an overlapping region for Δth dimension, $\delta_{old} - \delta_{new} > 0$ during the overlap test, hyperbox contraction is needed. Thus, during this condition, $\Delta = i$ and $\delta_{old} = \delta_{new}$. The test proceeds similarly to check other dimensions. If no overlapping region is found, Δ is set to -1 and the test stops indicating the contraction step is not required. Here, following cases are examined to determine the need for contraction based on hyperbox overlap test.

- Case 1

$$P_{j\Delta} < P_{k\Delta} < Q_{j\Delta} < Q_{k\Delta}, \quad Q_{j\Delta}^{new} = P_{k\Delta}^{new} = \frac{Q_{j\Delta}^{old} + P_{k\Delta}^{old}}{2} \tag{5.31}$$

- Case 2

$$P_{k\Delta} < P_{j\Delta} < Q_{k\Delta} < Q_{j\Delta}, \quad Q_{k\Delta}^{new} = P_{j\Delta}^{new} = \frac{Q_{k\Delta}^{old} + P_{j\Delta}^{old}}{2} \tag{5.32}$$

- Case 3

$$P_{j\Delta} = P_{k\Delta} < Q_{j\Delta} < Q_{k\Delta}, \qquad P_{k\Delta}^{new} = Q_{j\Delta}^{old} \tag{5.33}$$

- Case 4

$$P_{j\Delta} < P_{k\Delta} < Q_{j\Delta} = Q_{k\Delta}, \qquad Q_{j\Delta}^{new} = P_{k\Delta}^{old} \tag{5.34}$$

- Case 5

$$P_{k\Delta} = P_{j\Delta} < Q_{k\Delta} < Q_{j\Delta}, \qquad P_{j\Delta}^{new} = Q_{k\Delta}^{old} \tag{5.35}$$

- Case 6

$$P_{k\Delta} < P_{j\Delta} < Q_{k\Delta} = Q_{j\Delta}, \qquad Q_{k\Delta}^{new} = P_{j\Delta}^{old} \tag{5.36}$$

- Case 7(a)

$$P_{j\Delta} < P_{k\Delta} \leq Q_{k\Delta} = Q_{j\Delta}, \& \ (Q_{k\Delta} - P_{j\Delta}) < (Q_{j\Delta} - P_{k\Delta})$$
$$P_{j\Delta}^{new} = Q_{k\Delta}^{old} \tag{5.37}$$

- Case 7(b)

$$P_{j\Delta} < P_{k\Delta} \leq Q_{k\Delta} = Q_{j\Delta}, \& \ (Q_{k\Delta} - P_{j\Delta}) > (Q_{j\Delta} - P_{k\Delta})$$
$$Q_{j\Delta}^{new} = P_{k\Delta}^{old} \tag{5.38}$$

- Case 8(a)

$$P_{k\Delta} < P_{j\Delta} \leq Q_{k\Delta} < Q_{j\Delta}, \& \ (Q_{k\Delta} - P_{j\Delta}) < (Q_{j\Delta} - P_{k\Delta})$$
$$Q_{k\Delta}^{new} = P_{j\Delta}^{old} \tag{5.39}$$

- Case 8(b)

$$P_{k\Delta} < P_{j\Delta} \leq Q_{k\Delta} < Q_{j\Delta}, \& \ (Q_{k\Delta} - P_{j\Delta}) > (Q_{j\Delta} - P_{k\Delta})$$
$$P_{k\Delta}^{new} = Q_{j\Delta}^{old} \tag{5.40}$$

- Case 9(a)

$$P_{j\Delta} = P_{k\Delta} < Q_{j\Delta} = Q_{k\Delta}, \qquad Q_{j\Delta}^{new} = P_{k\Delta}^{new} = \frac{Q_{j\Delta}^{old} + P_{k\Delta}^{old}}{2} \tag{5.41}$$

- Case 9(b)

$$P_{k\Delta} = P_{j\Delta} < Q_{k\Delta} = Q_{j\Delta}, \quad Q_{k\Delta}^{new} = P_{j\Delta}^{new} = \frac{Q_{k\Delta}^{old} + P_{j\Delta}^{old}}{2} \quad (5.42)$$

The overview of the entire EFMMNN classifier algorithm for retinal vessel segmentation is summarized in pseudocode as Algorithm 5.1.

$Input = F_h$
$Hyperbox = B_j$
$B_j = (F_h, p_j, q_j, f(F_h, p_j, q_j)) \ \forall \ F_h \in I^n$
if $Max_n(Q_{ji}, f_{hi}) - Min_n(P_{ji}, f_{hi}) \leq \Theta$ **then**
$\quad |$ *Hyperbox Expansion*
else
$\quad |$ *New Hyperbox Formed*
end
Hyperbox Overlap Test
if $(\Delta = i \ \& \ \delta_{old} = \delta_{new})$ **then**
$\quad |$ *Overlap True*
$\quad |$ *Go to Loop*
else if $\Delta = -1$ **then**
$\quad |$ *No Overlap*
else

end
Loop: Hyperbox Contraction (Nine Cases)
if $O_k \leftarrow b_j$ **then**
$\quad | \quad 1 \leftarrow u_{jk}$
else
$\quad | \quad 0 \leftarrow u_{jk}$
end
$Output = U$

Algorithm 5.1: Pseudocode for EFMMNN Classifier

The 11-D feature vector is fed as input pattern to first node of EFMMNN classifier to obtain a two class binary output. The two factors primarily affect the performance of EFMMNN classifier i.e. Θ and nature of training data. If the similar data belongs to two different classes, the training recognition rate falls down. Moreover, the training data should be the best possible representative of the complete dataset available. Thus, the similar characteristic of training as well as test data helps in the exact formation of decision boundaries between two classes with the inclusion of input pattern in its hyperboxes. As value of Θ increases, hyperbox nodes and training time reduces and so the network complexity. But an increased Θ may lead to overlapping of hyperboxes and thus the increased misclassification rate. So an optimum value of Θ needs to be found. Θ was varied in the range of $0.15 \leq \Theta \leq 0.35$ and the no. of hyperboxes were found as illustrated in Table 5.1. It is experimentally observed that $\Theta = 0.25$ leads to highest accuracy in testing phase. The enhanced FMMNN have been used as a classifier, with the same proposed modified rules as in [130]. The required no. of hyperboxes with an optimum value of Θ have been found for the maximum and efficient extraction of retinal vessels.

TABLE 5.1: No. of hyperboxes obtained w.r.t. Θ

Θ	No. of Hyperboxes
0.15	1231
0.25	842
0.35	769

5.5 Results & Discussion

The section discusses the datasets, parameter settings and performance metrics involved during the evaluation of the proposed approach. The simplicity and effectiveness of fuzzy hyperbox classifier yields effective results altogether compete other existing supervised learning approaches.

5.5.1 Material

The method has been evaluated on two publicly available databases DRIVE [71] and STARE [102]. DRIVE database was formed as a result of retinopathy screening program held in The Netherlands. This database consists of 40 images, divided into 20 test and 20 training images. The manually segmented images as ground truth by experienced ophthalmologists are available for test set along with this database. The classifier is trained on 20 training images using 180000 pixel samples in such a way that 9000 pixels are chosen randomly from each image. The STARE database consists of 20 images, and there is no division of test and training set in particular. The 9000 pixels are randomly chosen from each image as like for DRIVE database to train the classifier on STARE dataset.

5.5.2 Parameter Settings

There has been use of various parameters during several steps in this approach. The parameters have been fixed based on contingent selection of image from DRIVE database. The same parameter values have been used for other images of DRIVE and STARE dataset without any alteration. Each parameter value used to attain the results is as listed in Table 5.2.

Difference of Gaussian highlights the edges present in the image. The two Gaussian profiles with differing variance are subtracted from each other to retain a band of frequencies that fall within area of interested edges. We have experimentally chosen $\sigma_2 = 1.4$ and $\sigma_1 = 1.0$. An optimum trade-off value of Strength (S) and Warp (W) reflects the vital edge information in phase stretch transform. A large value of W, results in addition of noise and added curvature in phase whereas a larger value of S, gives a better noise performance but a lower spatial resolution [131]. Thus, experimentally it is found that $S = 0.75$ and $W = 25$ extract the edge information with acceptable accuracy. The cut-off fraction c of 0.4 and gain parameter $\gamma_{PC} = 10$ are found to give sensible results for the given application. σ_x and σ_y are the standard deviation of Gabor envelope in x and y directions, respectively. $\sigma_x = 5$ and $\sigma_y = 1.25$ approximates the Gaussian envelope of Gabor to the profile of vessel. Bottom hat transformation is performed at multi-scales and multi-orientation. Six scales have been used in the range from 3-23 with the step of four as the vessel pixel width approximately fall in the corresponding range.

The resulting neural network is a three layered structure comprising first input layer of 11 nodes i.e no. of features, the second hidden layer consisting of 842 nodes i.e. no. of hyperboxes formed for the chosen Θ. The output layer has two nodes, each node corresponds to a binary class.

TABLE 5.2: Parameter values used during the proposed approach

Parameter	Value
σ_2	1.4
σ_1	1.0
S	0.75
W	25.00
T_θ	2.5
c	0.4
γ_{PC}	10
Λ	10
σ_x	5
σ_y	1.25
Θ	0.25
γ	40

5.5.3 Evaluation

The results of vessel segmentation are compared pixel wise with the available groundtruth database. There is either a correct determination of vessel pixel or false one. The four conditions to decide the classification measure are as given in Table 5.3. These four instances are formulated as confusion matrix for the respective DRIVE and STARE datasets as shown in the Table 5.4 and Table 5.5. The efficiency of the algorithm is determined by certain performance measures like sensitivity (Se), specificity (Sp) and accuracy (Acc) [11] specified in Table 5.6.

TABLE 5.3: Classification measure

	Groundtruth	
	Vessel pixels	Background pixels
Predicted Vessel Pixels	True positive (TP)	False positive (FP)
Predicted Background pixels	False negative (FN)	True negative (TN)

TABLE 5.4: Confusion matrix for DRIVE dataset

Total Pixels	Vessel pixels	Background pixels
Predicted Vessel Pixels	431879 (TP)	132018 (FP)
Predicted Background pixels	146066 (FN)	5889507 (TN)

TABLE 5.5: Confusion matrix for STARE dataset

Total Pixels	Vessel pixels	Background pixels
Predicted Vessel Pixels	480756 (TP)	226331 (FP)
Predicted Background pixels	163297 (FN)	7599619 (TN)

TABLE 5.6: Performance measure

Performance Measure	Formula
Se	$TP/(TP+FN)$
Sp	$TN/(TN+FP)$
Acc	$(TP+TN)/(TP+FP+TN+FN)$

Table 5.7 and Table 5.8 illustrates the image wise performance of the proposed algorithm on the DRIVE and STARE dataset, respectively. The average performance measures Acc, Se, Sp are 95.73%, 74.75% and 97.81% on DRIVE database and 95.51%, 74.65% and 97.11% on STARE database, respectively. Table 5.9 and Table 5.10 gives an comparison on DRIVE and STARE dataset, respectively, with the following supervised classification methods reported in literature: Staal t al. [72], Soares et al. [73], Ricci and Perfetti [74], You et al. [76], Marin et al. [77], Vega et al. [79], Fraz et al. [78], Roychowdhary et al. [81] , Zhu et al. [82]. The values of Se, Sp, Acc and time mentioned for the stated approaches are presented as stated by their authors for the respective datasets.

5.5.4   Discussion

A comparison of the proposed results with other supervised approaches present in the literature is briefed in Table 5.9 and Table 5.10 for DRIVE and STARE datasets, respectively. The comparison table reveals that the method proposed by Ricci and Perfetti [74] attains higher sensitivity on DRIVE database but the presence of pathological images in STARE dataset affects its performance in terms of specificity. Moreover, the absence of measure of segmentation time is an added limitation to the approach. The method proposed by Roychowdhary et al. [81] outperform on STARE database but shows a comparative lower performance on DRIVE dataset. When the results are jointly evaluated considering all the performance measures, the proposed approach provides the best performance than other existing methods on DRIVE database, being competitive to the performance of other segmentation algorithms on STARE database. The best results are highlighted in Table 5.9 and Table 5.10. Further, the total time required for segmentation of a single image is less than half a minute, running on a PC with an Intel(R) Corei5 7th Gen CPU at 2.50 GHz and 4 GB of RAM. The time required to segment a DRIVE image is approximately 12 seconds whereas for STARE image is nearly 18 seconds. The segmentation time is measure of time required to extract the retinal vessels from an RGB retinal image. The time requirement for segmentation of image in our proposed approach is less than the existing approaches in literature except as in [81]. Though the time required is few seconds more than [81], the proposed approach performs competitive in several other measures. The overall performance of our proposed, as demonstrated in Table 5.9 and Table 5.10 is surely beneficial in automated retinal vessel segmentation. The simplicity and effectiveness of fuzzy hyperbox classifier is an added advantage to the approach. The results altogether are effective and compete other existing approaches.

5.6   Chapter Summary

Accurate segmentation of vessels holds a noteworthy role in determining the progression of future risks involved in DR. This chapter is an attempt to propose an algorithm for efficient segmentation of retinal vessels with the help of recent computer vision techniques. An optimal 11-d feature vector, in which each feature is selected with reference to the properties and appearance of vessel is formed as a representation of the retinal vessels. The binary classification is carried out with the help of hyperbox based enhanced fuzzy min max neural network. This hyperbox classifier has several advantages over other supervised classifiers which are

TABLE 5.7: Individual imagewise result on DRIVE dataset

Image No.	Sensitivity	Specificity	Accuracy
1	83.88	96.87	95.71
2	75.07	98.48	96.08
3	72.88	96.93	94.53
4	74.03	98.17	95.95
5	72.10	98.62	96.14
6	72.25	97.33	94.90
7	70.73	98.32	95.80
8	67.53	97.45	95.08
9	63.80	98.78	95.92
10	75.08	97.84	95.95
11	73.90	98.01	95.86
12	75.41	97.81	95.88
13	70.46	98.03	95.33
14	78.49	97.56	96.02
15	83.36	96.71	95.75
16	77.60	98.18	96.07
17	67.51	98.16	95.57
18	76.11	97.83	96.11
19	87.61	97.45	95.72
20	77.37	97.74	96.24
Average	**74.76**	**97.81**	**95.73**

briefed in chapter. The algorithm is validated on two publicly available datasets DRIVE and STARE. The performance of the algorithm excels the state-of-the-art supervised learning algorithms presented in the literature. The presented approach will surely assist ophthalmologists in effective, easy and quick segmentation of retinal vessels.

TABLE 5.8: Individual imagewise result on STARE dataset

Image No.	Sensitivity	Specificity	Accuracy
1	65.96	96.55	93.23
2	73.57	95.37	96.04
3	71.45	95.38	93.95
4	67.48	98.58	97.39
5	68.48	95.92	93.44
6	72.26	97.00	95.28
7	84.76	96.77	95.81
8	85.64	96.21	95.42
9	81.39	97.06	95.83
10	75.44	96.74	95.02
11	86.45	97.17	96.41
12	86.01	97.95	97.02
13	74.03	98.00	95.87
14	72.52	97.73	95.44
15	64.14	97.45	94.57
16	62.50	97.29	93.74
17	85.34	96.63	95.62
18	69.68	98.51	96.55
19	71.97	98.48	96.04
20	73.86	97.34	97.41
Average	**74.65**	**97.11**	**95.51**

TABLE 5.9: Comparative analysis of the supervised learning based state-of-the-art methods on DRIVE dataset

Type	Method	Sensitivity	Specificity	Accuracy	Time
	2nd Human Observer	77.96	97.17	94.70	
Supervised Methods	Staal et al. [72]	71.9	97.7	94.4	900 s
	Soares et al. [73]	73.3	97.8	94.6	180 s
	Ricci and Perfetti [74]	77.5	97.2	95.9	-
	You et al. [76]	74.10	97.51	94.34	-
	Marin et al. [77]	70.67	98.01	94.52	~90 s
	Vega et al. [79]	74.44	96.00	94.12	-
	Fraz et al. [78]	74	98.1	94.8	~100 s
	Roychowdhary et al. [81]	72.5	98.3	95.2	~4 s
	Zhu et al. [82]	71.4	98.68	96.07	~12 s
	Proposed Method	**74.76**	**97.81**	**95.732**	**~12 s**

TABLE 5.10: Comparative analysis of the supervised learning based state-of-the-art methods on STARE dataset

Type	Method	Sensitivity	Specificity	Accuracy	Time
	2nd Human Observer	89.51	93.84	93.48	
Supervised Methods	Staal et al. [72]	69.7	98.1	95.2	900 s
	Soares et al. [73]	72	97.5	94.8	180 s
	Ricci and Perfetti [74]	90.3	93.9	96.5	-
	You et al. [76]	72.60	97.56	94.97	-
	Marin et al. [77]	69.44	98.19	95.26	~90 s
	Vega et al. [79]	70.19	96.71	94.83	-
	Fraz et al. [78]	75.5	97.6	95.3	~100 s
	Roychowdhary et al. [81]	**77.2**	**97.3**	**95.3**	**~7 s**
	Proposed Method	74.65	97.11	95.51	~18 s

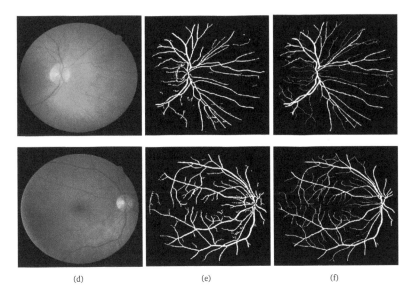

(d)   (e)   (f)

FIGURE 5.5: Results of proposed vessel segmentation on random images of DRIVE dataset: Column-wise (a) RGB Image, (b) Groundtruth Image, (c) Proposed vessel segmentation output Image

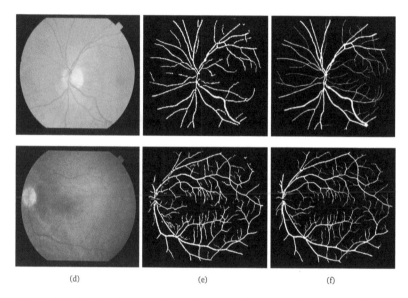

(d)   (e)   (f)

FIGURE 5.6: Results of proposed vessel segmentation on random images of STARE dataset : Column-wise (a) RGB Image, (b) Groundtruth Image, (c) Proposed vessel segmentation output Image

Chapter 6

Exploiting transfer learning using CBAM-U-Net for efficient retinal vessel segmentation

6.1 Introduction

DR causes damage to blood-retinal barrier which may lead to the abruption of vessels and leakage of blood onto retinal surface. The early indicators of DR at this stage are MA, HE, EX and SE. The advance stages include the proliferation of new blood vessels and also may lead to retinal detachment. Thus, the segmentation of blood vessels is important factor when screening the several stages of DR. It also plays a key role in retinal image registration. The retinal vessel extraction is a challenging task due to uneven intensity distribution, complex structure of subtle and tiny vessels, image distortion and artefacts included during its capture and several other imaging conditions.

Wide research has been carried out in finding techniques and algorithms to extract the vessels from retina images. Supervised and unsupervised learning techniques broadly classify the algorithms in two classes. Supervised approach is rule based learning with the help of manually labelled ground truth images also termed as gold standard. Unsupervised methods have no labelled samples in prior. It is evident from the machine learning and computer vision research, the immense feat is so far driven by supervised learning. The recent advancements in Deep Learning (DL) are 'Cherry on the Cake' for supervised learning. DL is expeditiously turning as avant-garde in medical image segmentation and have brought in excellent improvement in performance of various health care applications.

6.2 Related Work

Wang et al. [136] proposed an algorithm which employed CNN as stratified feature extractor and random forest leverages these learned features followed by ensemble learning. Fu et al. [84] exploited fully convolutional neural network derived from holistically-nested edge detection (HED) problem to generate vessel probability map. The similar kind of CNN approach for extracting retinal vessels is proposed by Hu et al. [85] at multi scales and Lisowski et al. [87] utilising structured prediction (SP).

CNN architectures are termed as fully convolutional when dense fully connected layers are removed [88]. Dasgupta and Singh [89] employed fully convolutional architecture for SP for retinal vessel segmentation. Sine-Net proposed by Atli and Gedik [90] cross connected CNN (CcNet) architecture by Feng et al. [91] used fully convolutional layers network to segment vessels. The transfer learning approach is used by Jiang et al. [92] which utilizes the pre-trained weights from AlexNet is presented in [88].

U-Net [93] serves as backbone in various medical image segmentation applications and have brought about a revolutionary change in the performance of semantic segmentation in particular. U-net, its several variants and flavours have contributed expeditiously in the application to segment vessels. Deformable U-Net (DU-Net) by Jin et al. [94], residual spatial attention network (RSAN) by Guo et al. [95], R2U-Net by Alom et al. [96], Dense-UNet by Guo et al. [98], BCDU-Net [97] obtained state-of-the-art performance in vessel segmentation.

As we mentioned, the immense success of machine learning has been a result of supervised learning. In this paper, we made an attempt to explore transfer learning (TL) for retinal vessel segmentation and we have attained at par performance.

During NIPS 2016 tutorial [137], Andrew Ng focused his talk on TL and stated that it will be the next driver of ML success after supervised learning. The opportunity to use the knowledge learned from the number of experiences and applying that to a new environment is the simple definition of TL.

The highlights of the proposed approach are as follows:

1. The TL phenomenon using DL networks has been exploited to increase the overall efficiency of retinal vessel segmentation algorithms.

2. The network is trained on DRIVE retinal image dataset and the weights of this network have been used to train the network with different retinal image datasets.

3. The TL network achieves an increased performance as compared to the network trained from scratch.

4. The training time required is less than what is needed to train the network from scratch and also the network attains excellent accuracy with small datasets and in small number of epochs.

5. The U-net [93] proposed by Ronneberger is utilised as a primary network with an added convolutional block attention module (CBAM) which results in increased representation power and thus improved performance of the network.

6.3 Methodology

6.3.1 Dataset Preparation

A simple yet effective pre-processing technique is applied to enhance the image equalisation and overall contrast of fundus image. The gray scale image encompasses the better information of retinal vessels and background, thus gray channel image is used for entire analysis. Data normalisation is applied as a part of data preparation which improves integrity of data and reduces redundancy. A tile based adaptive histogram equalisation CLAHE is applied which enhances the image while keeping the contrast in certain limits gives a final pre-processed image.

The number of training images in the available datasets with groundtruth are limited. Though U-Net gets trained on limited data, still to increase the accuracy of network and importantly to solve the issue of over-fitting, we increase the training data by randomly extracting the patches from the images. We extract the patch of size 64 × 64 from the available datasets with a specific condition that the patch includes the field of view (FOV) region. The entire black patch adds to class imbalance, thus the presence of more or less FOV region is the criteria held for sampling patches. The network is evaluated by distributing the datasets into training set, validation set and testing set. There are several ways to divide data into training and test sets. DRIVE [71] dataset consist of pre-defined 20 training images and the rest 20 images for testing. We adopted the same technique of random split of datasets into equal number of training and test images for STARE [102] and CHASE [78] datasets to avoid being biased towards any characteristics of data. Thus, STARE and CHASE datasets were trained and tested on 10 and 14 images each respectively. HRF [113] dataset has 45 images (15 each for healthy, DR and glaucoma), we formed a training set of 15 images by randomly choosing 5 images from each set.

6.3.2 CBAM-U-Net

Inspired by performance of U-Net and smooth integration of CBAM in any CNN architecture, we proposed CBAM-U-Net to segment retinal vessels. The proposed network has a similar encoder and decoder as like U-net with an additional attention module at bottleneck as shown in Figure 6.1. The module learns what and where to incite and inhibit and thus adds to refinement of representation power of the network. The addition of module leads to an increase in overall accuracy of the system without much increase in the parameters and training time. The dilated convolution also termed as atrous convolution with a dilation rate = 2 have been employed to increase the receptive field of convolution.

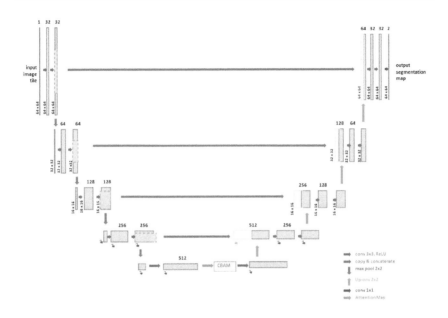

FIGURE 6.1: CBAM-U-Net architecture with image input tile of size 64×64

6.3.2.1 Basic U-Net

The task to extract retinal vessels falls under semantic segmentation i.e., classifying the label for each pixel within an image. The semantic segmentation was prominently explored based on fully convolutional networks in [88]. Further improvements to the approach in [88], is proposed by Ronnerberger in [93]. U-Net was developed by Ronnerberger et al. [93] specifically for Biomedical Image Segmentation. The network consists of two paths: encoder and decoder, which gives the network a U-shape and thus its name. The encoder path is a typical convolutional network that consists of stack of convolutions, each followed by a rectified linear unit (ReLU) activation and a max pooling operation. The encoder enhances the feature information whereas reduces the spatial information. The special aspect of this architecture is its expansion path i.e., decoder. After the contraction path, the grid size is expanded through a series of up-convolutions and upsampling to get the output image of the same size as input. The decoder pathway combines the high-resolution feature as well as spatial information from the contracting path which allow the network to propagate context information to higher resolution layers.

6.3.2.2 Convolutional Block Attention Module

Attention module have been incorporated in DL networks as it guides to focus on subject of interest and also improves the representation of interests. CBAM [138] consist of two attention modules viz. 'channel' and 'spatial' sequentially arranged one after the other. The channel attention focuses on 'what' is meaningful given an input feature and spatial attention focuses on 'where' is information of interest, which is contrary to channel attention. Thus, a sequential arrangement of these models helps to exploit both 'what' and 'where' in the feature map and improves the representation power of CNN network. The diagrammatic representation of CBAM module is as given in Figure 6.2

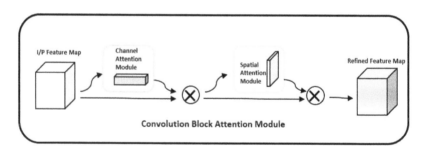

FIGURE 6.2: Convolutional Block Attention Module (CBAM)

Provided a input feature map $\mathbf{F} \in \mathbb{R}^{C \times H \times W}$, the sequential channel attention map $\mathbf{A_c} \in \mathbb{R}^{C \times 1 \times 1}$ and spatial attention map $\mathbf{A_s} \in \mathbb{R}^{1 \times H \times W}$ of CBAM module is as briefed in Figure 6.2. The final attention process output $\mathbf{F}_s$ is summarized as

$$\mathbf{F}_c = \mathbf{A_c}(\mathbf{F}) \otimes \mathbf{F}$$

$$\mathbf{F}_s = \mathbf{A_s}(\mathbf{F}_c) \otimes \mathbf{F}_c$$

Each module is individually illustrated as follows:

Channel-attention module:

A channel-attention module is created by leveraging the inter-channel relation between features. At the start, average pooled features $\mathbf{F}_{avg}^c$ and max-pooled features $\mathbf{F}_{max}^c$ are both generated to gather spatial information and distinct object features effectively. These feature descriptors are forwarded to a multi layer perceptron (MLP) with one hidden layer. The MLP weights $\mathbf{W_0} \in \mathbb{R}^{C/r \times C}$ and $\mathbf{W_1} \in \mathbb{R}^{C \times C/r}$ are shared for both the descriptors. A reduction ratio $r = 8$ is used for the application to reduce the parameter overhead and thus size of hidden activation is $\mathbb{R}^{C/r \times 1 \times 1}$. The output feature vector is combined through summation followed by a sigmoid activation function. Thus, the channel-attention is computed as follows:

$$\mathbf{A_c}(\mathbf{F}) = \sigma\left(\mathbf{W}_1\left(\mathbf{W}_0\left(\mathbf{F}_{\mathrm{avg}}^c\right)\right) + \mathbf{W}_1\left(\mathbf{W}_0\left(\mathbf{F}_{\mathrm{max}}^c\right)\right)\right)$$

Spatial-attention module:

A spatial-attention module is created by leveraging the inter-spatial relation between features. The average pooled features $\mathbf{F}_{avg}^s$ and max-pooled features $\mathbf{F}_{max}^s$ are generated along the channel axis, which results in emphasizing informative regions. These feature descriptors are then concatenated followed by a convolutional layer with filter size 7×7 to produce a 2-D spatial attention map. The sigmoid activation function σ applied thereafter gives the spatial-attention map as follows:

$$\mathbf{A_s}(\mathbf{F}) = \sigma\left(f^{7 \times 7}\left(\left[\mathbf{F}_{\mathbf{avg}}^{\mathbf{s}}; \mathbf{F}_{\mathbf{max}}^{\mathbf{s}}\right]\right)\right)$$

The step-wise illustration of each attention module is described in Figure 6.3.

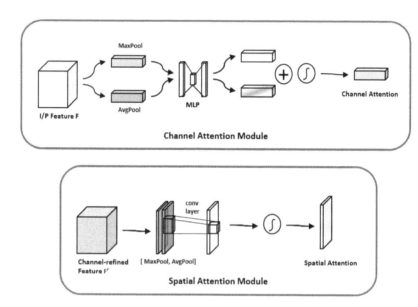

FIGURE 6.3: Individual Channel-attention module & Spatial-attention module

6.3.3 Transfer Learning

The transfer of knowledge from an environment to a new one is normally termed as transfer learning (TL). On similar terms, the application of knowledge of pre-trained CNN model on a related kind of problem is TL in DL. CNN yield the high performance as compared to several other machine learning algorithms but the requirement of bulk data and higher training time are the added limitations. The TL phenomenon comes to the rescue of these limitation with generally an added performance. The best possible use of knowledge of pre-trained model to a newer network does not require to train the network from scratch, thus require less training time as well as training data. But also TL is not a fixture to all kind of cases and problem. It attains the high performance only when it is appropriately suited and typically requires experimentation to find out its best pertinence.

There are several approaches while using TL on DL problems.

1. Training a model to reuse it

   A certain model trained for a task A with abundance of data can be reused to solve the task B which is not having enough training data. The use of entire model or only few layers or only change in task-specific output layers of the previous network, are the several options to work on depending upon the related problem.

2. Using a pre-trained model

   There are several pre-trained models available (GoogleNet, ResNet, VGG) which can be used for transfer learning, fine tuning and feature extraction. This approach is commonly used in deep learning depending upon the problem. The few fine modifications in usage of the pre-trained network layers can lead to excellent results in less training time.

3. Representation Learning

   This approach is also termed as feature extraction. The finding of important and relevant combination of features which are best representation of your problem from the CNN model is the purpose of this approach. DL models automatically extract features from raw image in a very quick timeframe, also for the complicated problems is a much-added advantage of this approach.

The unified definition of transfer learning [139] is given as follows: Given a source domain D_S and target domain D_T where $D = \{X, P(X)\}$ with respective source task T_S and target task T_T where $T = \{Y, P(Y|X)\}$. TL is defined as use of learned knowledge in D_S and T_S, to enhance the learning of target predictive function in D_T, where $D_S \neq D_T$ or $T_S \neq T_T$. Here X is the data instance and Y is the label associated with it. $P(X)$ is the marginal probability distribution and $P(Y|X)$ is conditional probability distribution.

With reference to our application, we are dealing with same feature spaces ($X_S = X_T$) and also same marginal probability distribution ($P(X_S) = P(X_T)$) as the application of vessel segmentation remains same. Thus, we have $D_S = D_T$. The vessel segmentation is a binary class problem and the source as well as target have equal number of classes to deal with, thus we have same label spaces ($Y_S = Y_T$). The difference lies in the conditional probability distribution $P(Y_S|X_S) \neq$

$P(Y_T|X_T)$, because the source and target datasets are different. The different distribution of classes in data makes the learning task different ($T_S \neq T_T$).

We opted an approach of training our proposed model to re-use its learned knowledge on the different retinal image datasets. We train our CBAM-U-Net on DRIVE dataset and reuse its best pre-trained weights to train the model on several different retinal datasets. Transfer learning is an optimization technique implemented either to save time or to attain improved performance. In retinal vessel segmentation, we achieved both these optimizations. The pre-trained weights make the network to get higher accuracy right from start and the network reaches to its highest accuracy in less training time as well as less number of epochs.

6.3.4   Performance Evaluation Metrics

The proposed model has been evaluated using several performance metrics namely sensitivity (SE), specificity (SP), precision (PR), accuracy (ACC), area under curve (AUC) of receiver operating characteristic (ROC). Accuracy is the measure of proportion of correctly classified pixels. Sensitivity is the measure of proportion of correctly classified positives whereas specificity is the measure of proportion of correctly classified negatives. Precision is the measure of correct positive predictions that actually belong to positive class. These metrics are computed as follows:

$$ACC = \frac{TP + TN}{TP + FP + TN + FN}$$

$$SE = \frac{TP}{TP + FN}$$

$$SP = \frac{TN}{TN + FP}$$

$$PR = \frac{TP}{TP + FP}$$

where TP is number of true positive samples, TN is number of true negative samples, FP represents number of false positive samples and FN is the number of false negative samples.

We also calculate F_1-score which is a measure of test's accuracy. It is harmonic mean of precision and recall (also called as sensitivity), stated as follows:

$$F_1 = 2 \cdot \frac{PR \cdot SE}{PR + SE}$$

6.4 Results & Discussion

The proposed model has been evaluated on the publicly available datasets DRIVE, STARE, CHASE, also including the high resolution fundus image dataset HRF briefed in Table 6.1. The data is split into training and test set as mentioned in Section 6.3.1. The Adam optimizer is used with a learning rate of 10^-5 for compiling the model. A dice co-efficient loss function is measure of overlap between two samples where 1 indicates perfect overlap. Our binary class problem of semantic segmentation attains maximum validation accuracy with the use of dice co-efficient loss function. The batch size of 16 is used to train and test the network with 30 training epochs. The proposed model has been initially trained from scratch on DRIVE dataset. The 64×64 size extracted patches from retinal image are the input to the proposed network and the same size output is achieved from the network. Figure 6.4 illustrated the randomly extracted patches and the corresponding groundtruth given as input to the proposed CBAM-U-Net. The segmentation results of DRIVE dataset for some random test images is presented in Figure 6.8.

6.4.1 Comparison against transfer learning

The another important aspect of proposed contribution is to exploit the benefits of employing TL to retinal vessel segmentation. Thus, the best weights of the trained network (on DRIVE dataset) are used as the pre-trained knowledge to train the

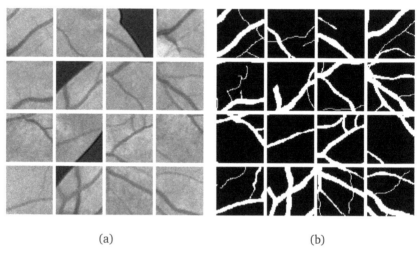

(a)   (b)

FIGURE 6.4: (a) 64×64 size training patches given as input to the CBAM-U-Net (b) Patches from the corresponding groundtruth

networks with retinal images of other datasets. The main aim of using TL is to save the time and have an advantage of the reliability of using tested models. The TL usually works for an application when it gives the benefits as like higher start, higher slope or higher asymptote on a graph of training v/s performance. Thus, we initially trained the network from scratch for STARE, CHASE and HRF datasets. Thereafter, the network was trained for these datasets using the pretrained knowledge of network trained on DRIVE dataset. Thus, we observed that the network trained using transfer learning attains higher start, higher slope and higher asymptote which is illustrated in Figure 6.5.

The performance of the model on the three datasets STARE, CHASE, HRF is evaluated for both the scenarios. Table 6.2 illustrates the segmentation results of the network trained from scratch and also after training the network using the pretrained weights of the network trained on DRIVE dataset. It reveals that the advent of transfer learning leads to an improvement in performance metrics for all the three datasets. Thus, the improved performance with less training time and less no. of epochs manifests the advantages of using TL for efficient retinal vessel segmentation. A ROC curve, is a graphical representation that illustrates the diagnostic ability of a system as its classification threshold is varied. AUC is area

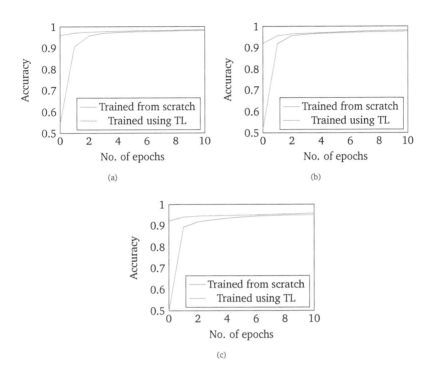

FIGURE 6.5: Comparison of training from scratch and training using pre-trained weights on (a) STARE (b) CHASE (c) HRF dataset

under the ROC curve which gives an aggregate measure of performance across all possible classification thresholds. AUC is calculated for each dataset and is illustrated in Figure 6.6. The ROC curve shows that the proposed network achieves excellent values of AUC and excels in performance. The segmentation results for some randomly selected images of STARE, CHASE, HRF datasets is as presented in Figure 6.9, Figure 6.10 and Figure 6.11 respectively. The illustrated image output is the result of the proposed network employed with TL on the respective datasets.

6.4.2 Comparison against existing DL methods

We have compared the performance of our network with the existing state-of-the-art deep learning methods for retinal vessel segmentation for DRIVE, STARE and CHASE datasets as briefed in Table 6.3. The DL approaches have outperformed the state-of-the-art approaches in a decade, thus we have made an extensive comparison with these methods.

The proposed network exhibits a competitive performance to the state-of-the-art methods. The method attains highest sensitivity and F_1 score on DRIVE dataset. The specificity of the transfer learning approach proposed by Jiang et al. [92] is higher than our approach, but it is at the cost of low sensitivity. Wang et al. [83] records a highest accuracy but the other performance metrics especially AUC is comparatively low. The approach by Jiang et al. [92] surpasses all other methods on STARE dataset, but the obtained metrics by proposed network are competitive. Our network excels performance on CHASE dataset. The approach by Jiang et al. [92] records higher sensitivity but at the cost of increased false positives. The specificity of SineNet of Atli and Gedik [90] is highest but they record too low sensitivity as compared to existing approaches. The proposed approach also excels in F_1 score on DRIVE and CHASE dataset. Very few DL architectures have been evaluated on HRF dataset due to its high resolution. The proposed network outperforms on HRF dataset when compared to the existing DL networks as illustrated in Table 6.3.

The proposed network extracts the vessel satisfactorily in challenging scenarios like low contrast vessels, tiny and thin vessels, vessels surrounding pathological area, vessel crossings and overlap. Figure 6.7 illustrates the randomly extracted patches comprising of several challenging scenarios along with the respective groundtruth and obtained output patches.

6.5 Conclusion

Deep neural networks have been extensively explored in the medical image segmentation. The U-net architecture in particular have laid the foundation of one of

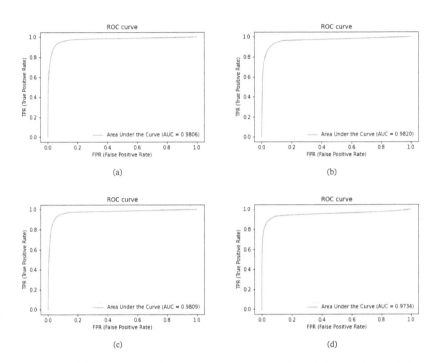

FIGURE 6.6: ROC Curve for the proposed network for (a) DRIVE dataset (b) STARE dataset (with TL) (c) CHASE dataset (with TL) (d) HRF dataset (with TL)

the best network to be employed for semantic segmentation. We have proposed this network by utilising the effective architecture of U-Net along with the attention module which holds a significant ability to increase the representation power of features of the network. CBAM acts as an important bottleneck component of the network and leads to an overall improved performance of in combination with U-Net. The seamless integration of CBAM to any CNN architecture with negligible overhead makes it more suitable and easy for use over other attention modules. The training of a deep neural network from scratch accompanies several constraints such as requirement of bulk training data, more number of epochs and training time to reach the maximum accuracy. The another important aspect of the proposed contribution is the employment of TF for retinal vessel segmentation. The use of learned knowledge of weights from DRIVE dataset during the training of networks on different retinal datasets shows a significant improvement in several aspects like training time, training epochs, validation accuracy and testing performance of the network. The concept of TL trains the network at ease and reaches improved accuracy in less number of data samples. The proposed approach is an attempt to showcase the future use of TL for the efficient retinal image analysis.

6.6 Chapter Summary

The chapter presented a DL architecture based CBAM-U-Net for semantic retinal vessel segmentation. The chapter also showcases the advantages of transfer learning for improved and efficient retinal vessel segmentation. An attention module CBAM is included at the bottleneck of U-Net architecture which results in refinement of classification by improving the representation of interest. The CBAM-U-Net is trained on the publicly available DRIVE dataset and this knowledge of this pre-trained network is used for training the network on different retinal image datasets. As the network need not be trained from scratch for these datasets, it attains the higher accuracies in lesser training time and less number of epochs. The transfer learning approach is validated on STARE, CHASE-DB1 and HRF datasets. The performance of the proposed approach excels the existing algorithms of vessel segmentation. The exploration of transfer learning and its performance provides an opportunity for its future potential use in retinal image analysis.

TABLE 6.1: Publicly available datasets used in the proposed approach

Dataset	Abbreviation	Image Source	Image Resolution	No. of Images	Healthy Images	Pathology Images
DRIVE	Digital Retinal Images for Vessel Extraction	Diabetic Retinopathy Screening Program, The Netherlands	565 × 584	20(Train) 20(Test)	33	07
STARE	STructured Analysis of the Retina	Shiley Eye Center University of California, San Diego. & The Veterans Administration Medical Center, San Diego	700 × 605	20	09	11
CHASE-DB1	Child Heart And Health Study in England	Kingston University London	999 × 960	28	28	00
HRF	High-Resolution Fundus	Pattern Recognition Lab, FAUEN (Germany) & The Brno University of Technology, Brno(Czech Republic)	3504 × 2336	45	15	15(DR) 15(Glaucoma)

TABLE 6.2: Comparison of performance metrics of proposed network on training with scratch and training using transfer learning

Database	Methods	Sensitivity	Specificity	Accuracy	AUC	F_1 Score
STARE	CBAM-U-Net	0.8141	0.9731	0.9585	0.9755	0.7830
	CBAM-U-Net (with TL)	0.8233	0.9833	0.9679	0.9820	0.8312
CHASE-DB1	CBAM-U-Net	0.8178	0.9792	0.9644	0.9809	0.8080
	CBAM-U-Net (with TL)	0.8312	0.9806	0.9671	0.9809	0.8206
HRF	CBAM-U-Net	0.7608	0.9906	0.96	0.9688	0.8353
	CBAM-U-Net (with TL)	0.7724	0.9920	0.9629	0.9734	0.8462

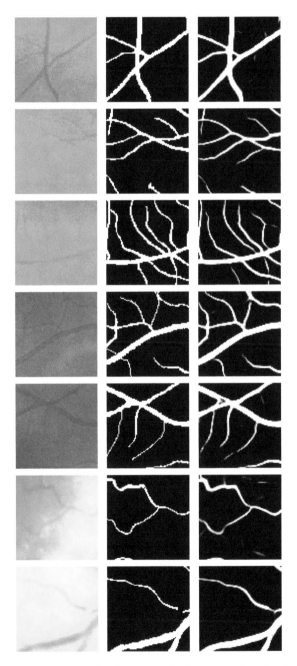

FIGURE 6.7: Column-wise: 1st Column : Randomly extracted patches from retinal images showcasing various challenging scenarios ; 2nd Column : Groundtruth for the corresponding input patches ; 3rd Column : Output of the proposed algorithm for the corresponding patches

TABLE 6.3: Comparative analysis of state-of-the-art deep learning approaches on different datasets

Database	Methods	Year	Sensitivity	Specificity	Accuracy	AUC	F_1 score
DRIVE	Wang et al.[83]	2014	0.8173	0.9733	0.9767	0.9475	-
	Li et al. [140]	2015	0.7569	0.9816	0.9527	0.9738	-
	Mo & Zhang [141]	2017	0.7779	0.9780	0.9521	0.9782	-
	Jiang et al. [92]	2018	0.7540	0.9825	0.9624	0.9810	-
	Hu et al. [85]	2018	0.7772	0.9793	0.9533	0.9759	-
	Alom et al. [96]	2018	0.7792	0.9813	0.9556	0.9784	0.8171
	Feng et al.[91]	2019	0.7625	0.9809	0.9528	0.9678	-
	Jin et al. [94]	2019	0.7963	0.9800	0.9566	0.9802	0.8237
	Azad et al. [97]	2019	0.8007	0.9786	0.9560	0.9789	0.8224
	Atli & Gedik [90]	2020	0.8260	0.9824	0.9685	0.9852	-
	Proposed	2021	0.8413	0.9802	0.9647	0.9806	0.8420
STARE	Wang et al. [83]	2014	0.8104	0.9791	0.9813	0.9751	-
	Li et al. [140]	2015	0.7726	0.9844	0.9628	0.9879	-
	Mo & Zhang [141]	2017	0.8147	0.9844	0.9674	0.9885	-
	Jiang et al. [92]	2018	0.8352	0.9846	0.9734	0.9900	-
	Hu et al. [85]	2018	0.7543	0.9814	0.9632	0.9751	-
	Alom et al. [96]	2018	0.8298	0.9862	0.9712	0.9914	0.8475
	Feng et al. [91]	2019	0.7709	0.9848	0.9633	0.9700	-
	Jin et al. [94]	2019	0.7595	0.9878	0.9641	0.9832	0.8143
	Atli & Gedik [90]	2020	0.6776	0.9946	0.9711	0.9807	-
	Proposed	2021	0.8233	0.9833	0.9679	0.9820	0.8312
CHASE-DB1	Li et al. [140]	2015	0.7507	0.9793	0.9581	0.9716	-
	Mo & Zhang [141]	2017	0.7661	0.9816	0.9599	0.9812	-
	Jiang et al. [92]	2018	0.8640	0.9745	0.9668	0.9810	-
	Alom et al. [96]	2018	0.7756	0.9820	0.9634	0.9815	0.7928
	Jin et al. [94]	2019	0.8155	0.9752	0.9610	0.9804	0.7883
	Atli & Gedik [90]	2020	0.7856	0.9845	0.9676	0.9828	-
	Proposed	2021	0.8312	0.9806	0.9671	0.9809	0.8206
HRF	Yan et al. [142]	2018	0.7881	0.9592	0.9437	-	-
	Jin et al. [94]	2019	0.7464	0.9874	0.9651	0.9831	-
	Proposed	2021	0.7724	0.9920	0.9629	0.9734	0.8462

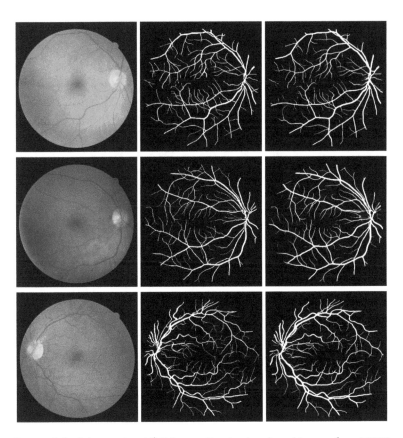

FIGURE 6.8: Column-wise: 1st Column : Randomly selected images from DRIVE dataset ; 2nd Column : Groundtruth for the corresponding input images ; 3rd Column : Output of the proposed algorithm for the corresponding images

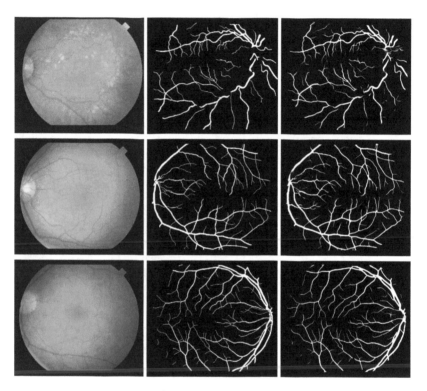

FIGURE 6.9: Column-wise: 1st Column : Randomly selected images from STARE dataset ; 2nd Column : Groundtruth for the corresponding input images ; 3rd Column : Output of the proposed algorithm for the corresponding images

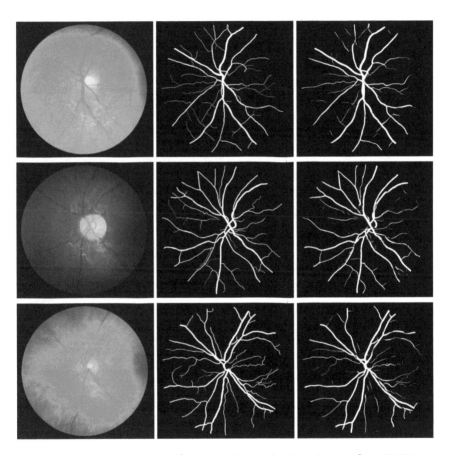

FIGURE 6.10: Column-wise: 1st Column : Randomly selected images from CHASE dataset ; 2nd Column : Groundtruth for the corresponding input images ; 3rd Column : Output of the proposed algorithm for the corresponding images

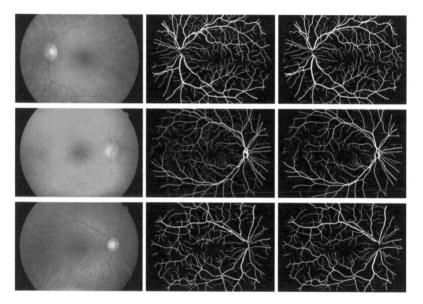

FIGURE 6.11: Column-wise: 1st Column : Randomly selected images from HRF dataset ; 2nd Column : Groundtruth for the corresponding input images ; 3rd Column : Output of the proposed algorithm for the corresponding images

Chapter 7

Conclusion and Future Scope

7.1 Conclusion

This thesis has presented novel techniques for information extraction from retinal fundus images. These efforts were aimed at contributing to the field of retinal image analysis for an effective screening of DR. The recent computer vision and machine learning techniques were utilized to extract the normal and abnormal features of retina in a way which could assist ophthalmologists in computer aided screening and diagnosis of DR. Firstly, a simple yet effective unsupervised algorithm was implemented to extract the white lesions i.e. exudates (EX). Secondly, we focussed on extracting the lesion which is an earliest indication of DR i.e. microaneurysms (MA). Accurate retinal segmentation is a pre-requisite during each stage of DR. Thus, we elaborated our thesis for efficient vessel segmentation in two different ways. The third contribution aimed at extracting retinal vessel by supervised fuzzy min max hyperbox based classification. The another contribution utilised the power of deep neural network and features of transfer learning for efficient and quick retinal vessel segmentation. All the proposed approaches are evaluated using the publicly available retinal datasets which are captured in several varying imaging conditions and are validated by retinal experts. The conclusions from four categories of contributions made in this thesis are as follows:

7.1.1 Exudate Detection

The proposed approach is a way to extract the EX in quick and easiest way. Though an unsupervised approach, the proposed algorithm has shown better results over other existing morphological image processing based methods. The introduction of K-means clustering algorithm along with the morphological method helps to find the lesions more effectively. The method attains a relatively greater sensitivity over other existing methods but it can be improved because the low intensity EX pixels are still too subtle to be detected by this algorithm. Our algorithm reaches high value of specificity which indicate that the detection of false positives is very less. This algorithm is an attempt to help the ophthalmologists in the DR screening process to detect EX from non-mydriatic low-contrast retinal digital images faster and more easily. The proposed method has obtained high values and sensitivity and specificity, and thus suitable for the screening of DR. The additional advantage of the proposed algorithm is it can be implemented very well even with a low configuration computing system.

7.1.2 MA Detection

A new approach for MA detection based on a set of invariant moment features and RUSBoost classifier have been proposed in this paper. Candidate extraction algorithm is employed to pre-processed image to detect the potential candidates. Invariant moment features are demonstrated as excellent MA shape descriptor along with shape and intensity features. Random undersampling adaboost classifier is employed to classify minority MA from spurious candidates. Although conventional supervised classification approach is used, the performance of the method strongly manifests its ability in real time automated screening of DR. The proposed method achieves significant performance on ROC and DIARETDB1 datasets as compared to existing MA detection techniques. The approach works satisfactorily on e-ophtha database. The method performs well in identifying low contrast and subtle MA. The future scope will concentrate on increasing the sensitivity of algorithm by utilising the suitable deep neural network architecture which do not require hand-crafted features and which could outperform on small datsets also.

7.1.3 Vessel Segmentation

The thesis includes two contribution for retinal vessel segmentation. It is a pre-requisite for NPDR as well as PDR screening, and also involves the various challenging aspects during its implementation. Firstly, a supervised retinal vessel extraction approach based on EFMMNN is attempted. An optimal short length 11-D feature vector consisting of spatial as well as frequency domain information is fed as input to the neural network. The hyperbox formation and its membership function is the distinct feature of this fuzzy based neural network. The online learning capability of the classifier without the need of any back propagation is essence of this neural network. The output of the classifier is binary and needs no further post processing. The method is evaluated on two datasets, DRIVE and STARE. The method utilizes only eleven features for pixel based classification, requires less computational time. The simplicity of the classifier used is an added advantage and needs to be highlighted. A three layered neural network without any need of back propagation algorithm outperforms the other existing supervised classification methods. Results of the proposed method in terms of Accuracy and Sensitivity are highly competitive and also performs well for pathological images as compared to existing supervised classification methodologies reported in literature. The method fails to extract very thin retinal vessels and the future work could be addressed to extract those well. The simplicity and effectiveness of the approach along with its fast implementation, makes this proposed method useful in computer aided vessel segmentation and screening for early detection of DR.

The supervised learning have been a foremost driver in the success of machine learning, and the future era aims at transfer learning to be the next driver. Thus, in our fourth contribution, we explored an approach to segment retinal vessels utilising the DL architecture and concept of transfer learning. This segmantic segmentation application is implemented using a CBAM-U-Net with the advantages of transfer learning. The bottleneck attention-module CBAM focuses on improving the feature representation power of the network, thus results in improved performance of U-Net. Moreover, the re-trained weights of CBAM-U-Net on DRIVE dataset have been utilised for training the network on another three publicly available datasets namely STARE, CHASE and HRF. The higher accuracy is attained in lesser training time, training data and number of epochs. The performance indices of the approach excels the state-of-the-art DL algorithms as well as supervised learning approaches.

7.2 Future Research Direction

There have been immense development in the area of retinal image analysis for screening of DR. Several researches have been carried out for CAD of DR and various drives are being carried to make use of this research in actual healthcare clinical practice. The recent DL architectures have boosted the performance of the screening algorithms and led to the new area of development. The new technological advances in computational power, machine learning methods and various cloud computing platforms provide biomedical scientists with an opportunity to drive automated models towards practical clinical potential. The detection of lesions and grading of DR has always been a cornerstone. The DL models could be explored more for segmentation of normal and abnormal structures of retina. The fuzzy min max neural network approach in the thesis can be extended for segmentation of lesions. The advantages of transfer learning along with DL could be explored even more to screen lesions efficiently and for disease severity grading.

The purpose of the techniques presented in this thesis was to identify anomalies in diabetic patients in early stages, that may lead to visual impairment in advance stages. However, future studies may be directed at improving strategies for detection of vessel width changes and neovascularization, which are the areas yet to get the focussed attention. In addition, the classification of arteries and veins, accurate measurement of widths and tortuosity that serve as an identifier for hypertensive retinopathy and cardiovascular risk factors, the vessel segmentation approaches could be broadened and explored.

Bibliography

[1] A. D. Association *et al.*, "Classification and diagnosis of diabetes: Standards of medical care in diabetes—2020," *Diabetes Care*, vol. 43, pp. S14–S31, 2020.

[2] Diabetes Atlas, "International Diabetes Federation, Brussels, Belgium," 2019.

[3] A. A. Alghadyan, "Diabetic retinopathy – an update," *Saudi Journal of Ophthalmology*, vol. 25, no. 2, pp. 99–111, 2011.

[4] ICO, "Guidelines for diabetic eye care, 2nd edn," *International Council of Ophthalmology (ICO)*, 2017.

[5] T. Y. Wong, C. M. G. Cheung, M. Larsen, S. Sharma, and R. Simó, "Diabetic retinopathy," *Nature Reviews Disease Primers*, 2016.

[6] C. Wilkinson, F. L. Ferris, R. E. Klein, P. P. Lee, C. D. Agardh, M. Davis, D. Dills, A. Kampik, R. Pararajasegaram, and J. T. Verdaguer, "Proposed international clinical diabetic retinopathy and diabetic macular edema disease severity scales," *Ophthalmology*, vol. 110, no. 9, pp. 1677–1682, 2003.

[7] R. Raman, L. Gella, S. Srinivasan, and T. Sharma, "Diabetic retinopathy: An epidemic at home and around the world," *Indian Journal of Ophthalmology*, vol. 64, no. 1, pp. 69–75, 2016.

[8] R. S. Eshaq, A. M. Aldalati, J. S. Alexander, and N. R. Harris, "Diabetic retinopathy: Breaking the barrier," *Pathophysiology*, vol. 24, no. 4, pp. 229–241, 2017.

[9] N. Patton, T. Aslam, T. MacGillivray, A. Pattie, I. J. Deary, and B. Dhillon, "Retinal vascular image analysis as a potential screening tool for cerebrovascular disease: a rationale based on homology between cerebral and retinal microvasculatures," *Journal of Anatomy*, vol. 206, no. 4, pp. 319–348, 2005.

[10] R. Winder, P. Morrow, I. McRitchie, J. Bailie, and P. Hart, "Algorithms for digital image processing in diabetic retinopathy," *Computerized Medical Imaging and Graphics*, vol. 33, no. 8, pp. 608–622, 2009.

[11] M. D. Abramoff, M. K. Garvin, and M. Sonka, "Retinal imaging and image analysis.," *IEEE Reviews in Biomedical Engineering*, vol. 3, pp. 169–208, 2010.

[12] K. C. Jordan, M. Menolotto, N. M. Bolster, I. A. Livingstone, and M. E. Giardini, "A review of feature-based retinal image analysis," *Expert Review of Ophthalmology*, vol. 12, no. 3, pp. 207–220, 2017.

[13] M. R. K. Mookiah, U. R. Acharya, C. K. Chua, C. M. Lim, E. Ng, and A. Laude, "Computer-aided diagnosis of diabetic retinopathy: A review," *Computers in Biology and Medicine*, vol. 43, no. 12, pp. 2136–2155, 2013.

[14] M. F. Nørgaard and J. Grauslund, "Automated screening for diabetic retinopathy–a systematic review," *Ophthalmic research*, vol. 60, no. 1, pp. 9–17, 2018.

[15] M. R. K. Mookiah, S. Hogg, T. J. MacGillivray, V. Prathiba, R. Pradeepa, V. Mohan, R. M. Anjana, A. S. Doney, C. N. Palmer, and E. Trucco, "A review of machine learning methods for retinal blood vessel segmentation and artery/vein classification," *Medical Image Analysis*, vol. 68, p. 101905, 2021.

[16] T. A. Soomro, A. J. Afifi, L. Zheng, S. Soomro, J. Gao, O. Hellwich, and M. Paul, "Deep learning models for retinal blood vessels segmentation: A review," *IEEE Access*, vol. 7, pp. 71696–71717, 2019.

[17] J. I. Orlando, E. Prokofyeva, M. del Fresno, and M. B. Blaschko, "An ensemble deep learning based approach for red lesion detection in fundus

images," *Computer Methods and Programs in Biomedicine*, vol. 153, pp. 115–127, 2018.

[18] P. Chudzik, S. Majumdar, F. Calivá, B. Al-Diri, and A. Hunter, "Microaneurysm detection using fully convolutional neural networks," *Computer Methods and Programs in Biomedicine*, vol. 158, pp. 185–192, 2018.

[19] W. Chen, B. Yang, J. Li, and J. Wang, "An approach to detecting diabetic retinopathy based on integrated shallow convolutional neural networks," *IEEE Access*, vol. 8, pp. 178552–178562, 2020.

[20] S. B. Rangrej and J. Sivaswamy, "Assistive lesion-emphasis system: an assistive system for fundus image readers," *Journal of Medical Imaging*, vol. 4, no. 2, p. 024503, 2017.

[21] D. Y. Carson Lam, M. Guo, and T. Lindsey, "Automated detection of diabetic retinopathy using deep learning," *AMIA Summits on Translational Science Proceedings*, vol. 2017, p. 147, 2018.

[22] M. M. Islam, H. C. Yang, T. N. Poly, W. S. Jian, and Y. C. Jack Li, "Deep learning algorithms for detection of diabetic retinopathy in retinal fundus photographs: A systematic review and meta-analysis," *Computer Methods and Programs in Biomedicine*, vol. 191, p. 105320, 2020.

[23] G. García, J. Gallardo, A. Mauricio, J. López, and C. Del Carpio, "Detection of diabetic retinopathy based on a convolutional neural network using retinal fundus images," in *International Conference on Artificial Neural Networks*, pp. 635–642, Springer, 2017.

[24] N. Tajbakhsh, J. Y. Shin, S. R. Gurudu, R. T. Hurst, C. B. Kendall, M. B. Gotway, and J. Liang, "Convolutional neural networks for medical image analysis: Full training or fine tuning?," *IEEE Transactions on Medical Imaging*, vol. 35, no. 5, pp. 1299–1312, 2016.

[25] V. Gulshan, L. Peng, M. Coram, M. C. Stumpe, D. Wu, A. Narayanaswamy, S. Venugopalan, K. Widner, T. Madams, J. Cuadros, *et al.*, "Development and validation of a deep learning algorithm for detection of diabetic retinopathy in retinal fundus photographs," *JAMA Ophthalmology*, vol. 316, no. 22, pp. 2402–2410, 2016.

[26] M. D. Abràmoff, Y. Lou, A. Erginay, W. Clarida, R. Amelon, J. C. Folk, and M. Niemeijer, "Improved automated detection of diabetic retinopathy on a publicly available dataset through integration of deep learning," *Investigative ophthalmology & visual science*, vol. 57, no. 13, pp. 5200–5206, 2016.

[27] G. Quellec, K. Charrière, Y. Boudi, B. Cochener, and M. Lamard, "Deep image mining for diabetic retinopathy screening," *Medical Image Analysis*, vol. 39, pp. 178–193, 2017.

[28] S. K. Lynch, A. Shah, J. C. Folk, X. Wu, and M. D. Abramoff, "Catastrophic failure in image-based convolutional neural network algorithms for detecting diabetic retinopathy," *Investigative Ophthalmology & Visual Science*, vol. 58, no. 8, p. 3776, 2017.

[29] T. Walter, J.-C. Klein, P. Massin, and A. Erginay, "A contribution of image processing to the diagnosis of diabetic retinopathy — detection of exudates in color fundus images of the human retina.," *IEEE Transactions on Medical Imaging*, vol. 21, no. 10, pp. 1236–1243, 2002.

[30] A. Sopharak, B. Uyyanonvara, and S. Barman, "Automatic detection of diabetic retinopathy exudates from non-dilated retinal images using mathematical morphology methods," *Computerized Medical Imaging and Graphics*, vol. 32, pp. 720–727, 2008.

[31] D. Welfer, J. Scharcanskia, and D. R. Marinho, "A coarse-to-fine strategy for automatically detecting exudates in color eye fundus images," *Computerized Medical Imaging and Graphics*, vol. 34, pp. 228–235, 2010.

[32] A. Sopharak, B. Uyyanonvara, and S. Barman, "Automatic exudate detection from non-dilated diabetic retinopathy retinal images using fuzzy c-means clustering," *Sensors ISSN 1424-8220.*, vol. 9, pp. 2148–2161, 2009.

[33] H. Yazid, H. Arof, and H. Mohd Isa, "Automated identification of exudates and optic disc based on inverse surface thresholding," *Journal of Medical Systems*, vol. 36, no. 3, pp. 1997–2004, 2012.

[34] G. G. Gardner, D. Keating, T. H. Williamson, and A. T. Elliott, "Automatic detection of diabetic retinopathy using an artificial neural network: a screening tool," *British Journal of Ophthalmology*, no. 80, pp. 940–944, 1996.

[35] M. Garcia, C. I. Sanchez, A. Mayo, M. I. Lopez, and R. Hornero, "Neural network based detection of hard exudates in retinal images," *Computer Methods and Programs in Biomedicine*, vol. 93, pp. 9–19, 2009.

[36] A. Osareh, B. Shadgar, and R. Markham, "A computational-intelligence-based approach for detection of exudates in diabetic retinopathy images," *IEEE Transaction on Information Technology in Biomedicine*, vol. 13, no. 4, pp. 535–545, 2009.

[37] H. Zhang and O. Chutatape, "Top-down and bottom-up strategies in lesion detection of background diabetic retinopathy.," *IEEE Computer Society Conference in Computer Vision and Pattern Recognition*, vol. 2, p. 422–428, 2005.

[38] G. Mahendran, R. Dhanasekaran, and K. N. Narmadha Devi, "Identification of exudates for diabetic retinopathy based on morphological process and pnn classifier," *International Conference on Communication and Signal Processing*, pp. 1117–1121, 2014.

[39] A. Osareh, M. Mirmehdi, B. Thomas, and R. Markham, "Comparative exudate classification using support vector machines and neural networks," *Springer Medical Image Computing and Computer-Assisted Intervention*, vol. 2489, p. 413–420, 2002.

[40] C. I. Sanchez, M. Garcia, A. Mayo, M. I. Lopez, and R. Hornero, "Retinal image analysis based on mixture models to detect hard exudates," *Medical Image Analysis*, vol. 13, no. 4, pp. 650–658, 2009.

[41] C. Sinthanayothin, J. F. Boyce, T. H. Williamson, H. L. Cook, E. Mensah, S. Lal, and D. Usher, "Automated detection of diabetic retinopathy on digital fundus images," *Diabetic Medicine*, vol. 19, no. 2, pp. 105–112, 2002.

[42] N. G. Ranamuka and R. G. N. Meegama, "Detection of hard exudates from diabetic retinopathy images using fuzzy logic," *Image Processing, IET*, vol. 7, no. 2, pp. 121–130, 2012.

[43] T. Walter, P. Massin, A. Erginay, R. Ordonez, C. Jeulin, and J.-C. Klein, "Automatic detection of microaneurysms in color fundus images," *Medical Image Analysis*, vol. 11, no. 6, pp. 555–566, 2007.

[44] M. Niemeijer, B. van Ginneken, J. Staal, M. S. A. Suttorp-Schulten, and M. D. Abramoff, "Automatic detection of red lesions in digital color fundus photographs," *IEEE Transactions on Medical Imaging*, vol. 24, pp. 584–592, May 2005.

[45] A. J. Frame, P. E. Undrill, M. J. Cree, J. A. Olson, K. C. McHardy, P. F. Sharp, and J. V. Forrester, "A comparison of computer based classification methods applied to the detection of microaneurysms in ophthalmic fluorescein angiograms," *Computers in Biology and Medicine*, vol. 28, no. 3, pp. 225–238, 1998.

[46] A. Mizutani, C. Muramatsu, Y. Hatanaka, S. Suemori, T. Hara, and H. Fujita, "Automated microaneurysm detection method based on double ring filter in retinal fundus images," *Proc.SPIE*, vol. 7260, pp. 7260 – 7260 – 8, 2009.

[47] C. I. Sanchez, R. Hornero, A. Mayo, and M. García, "Mixture model-based clustering and logistic regression for automatic detection of microaneurysms in retinal images," *Proc.SPIE*, vol. 7260, pp. 7260 – 7260 – 8, 2009.

[48] B. Zhang, X. Wu, J. You, Q. Li, and F. Karray, "Detection of microaneurysms using multi-scale correlation coefficients," *Pattern Recognition*, vol. 43, no. 6, pp. 2237–2248, 2010.

[49] B. Zhang, F. Karray, Q. Li, and L. Zhang, "Sparse representation classifier for microaneurysm detection and retinal blood vessel extraction," *Information Sciences*, vol. 200, pp. 78–90, 2012.

[50] G. Quellec, M. Lamard, P. M. Josselin, G. Cazuguel, B. Cochener, and C. Roux, "Optimal wavelet transform for the detection of microaneurysms in retina photographs," *IEEE Transactions on Medical Imaging*, vol. 27, pp. 1230–1241, Sept 2008.

[51] K. Ram, G. D. Joshi, and J. Sivaswamy, "A successive clutter-rejection-based approach for early detection of diabetic retinopathy," *IEEE Transactions on Biomedical Engineering*, vol. 58, pp. 664–673, March 2011.

[52] L. Giancardo, F. Meriaudeau, T. P. Karnowski, Y. Li, K. W. Tobin, and E. Chaum, "Microaneurysm detection with radon transform-based classification on retina images," in *2011 Annual International Conference of the IEEE Engineering in Medicine and Biology Society*, pp. 5939–5942, Aug 2011.

[53] B. Antal and A. Hajdu, "An ensemble-based system for microaneurysm detection and diabetic retinopathy grading," *IEEE Transactions on Biomedical Engineering*, vol. 59, pp. 1720–1726, June 2012.

[54] I. Lazar and A. Hajdu, "Retinal microaneurysm detection through local rotating cross-section profile analysis," *IEEE Transactions on Medical Imaging*, vol. 32, pp. 400–407, Feb 2013.

[55] M. U. Akram, S. Khalid, A. Tariq, S. A. Khan, and F. Azam, "Detection and classification of retinal lesions for grading of diabetic retinopathy," *Computers in Biology and Medicine*, vol. 45, pp. 161–171, 2014.

[56] K. M. Adal, D. Sidibé, S. Ali, E. Chaum, T. P. Karnowski, and F. Mériaudeau, "Automated detection of microaneurysms using scale-adapted blob analysis and semi-supervised learning," *Computer Methods and Programs in Biomedicine*, vol. 114, no. 1, pp. 1–10, 2014.

[57] B. Dai, X. Wu, and W. Bu, "Retinal microaneurysms detection using gradient vector analysis and class imbalance classification," *PLOS ONE*, vol. 11, no. 8, pp. 1–23, 2016.

[58] L. Seoud, T. Hurtut, J. Chelbi, F. Cheriet, and J. M. P. Langlois, "Red lesion detection using dynamic shape features for diabetic retinopathy screening," *IEEE Transactions on Medical Imaging*, vol. 35, pp. 1116–1126, April 2016.

[59] S. A. A. Shah, A. Laude, I. Faye, and T. B. Tang, "Automated microaneurysm detection in diabetic retinopathy using curvelet transform," *Journal of Biomedical Optics*, vol. 21, no. 10, pp. 1–8, 2016.

[60] B. Wu, W. Zhu, F. Shi, S. Zhu, and X. Chen, "Automatic detection of microaneurysms in retinal fundus images," *Computerized Medical Imaging and Graphics (Special Issue on Ophthalmic Medical Image Analysis)*, vol. 55, pp. 106–112, 2017.

[61] S. Wang, H. L. Tang, L. I. A. turk, Y. Hu, S. Sanei, G. M. Saleh, and T. Peto, "Localizing microaneurysms in fundus images through singular spectrum analysis," *IEEE Transactions on Biomedical Engineering*, vol. 64, pp. 990–1002, May 2017.

[62] S. S. Kar and S. P. Maity, "Automatic detection of retinal lesions for screening of diabetic retinopathy," *IEEE Transactions on Biomedical Engineering*, vol. 65, pp. 608–618, March 2018.

[63] F. Ren, P. Cao, W. Li, D. Zhao, and O. Zaiane, "Ensemble based adaptive over-sampling method for imbalanced data learning in computer aided detection of microaneurysm," *Computerized Medical Imaging and Graphics*, vol. 55, pp. 54–67, 2017.

[64] W. Zhou, C. Wu, D. Chen, Y. Yi, and W. Du, "Automatic microaneurysm detection using the sparse principal component analysis-based unsupervised classification method," *IEEE Access*, vol. 5, pp. 2563–2572, 2017.

[65] B. Dashtbozorg, J. Zhang, F. Huang, and B. M. ter Haar Romeny, "Retinal microaneurysms detection using local convergence index features," *IEEE Transactions on Image Processing*, vol. 27, no. 7, pp. 3300–3315, 2018.

[66] W. Cao, N. Czarnek, J. Shan, and L. Li, "Microaneurysm detection using principal component analysis and machine learning methods," *IEEE Transactions on NanoBioscience*, vol. 17, pp. 191–198, July 2018.

[67] V. Deepa, C. Sathish Kumar, and S. Susan Andrews, "Automated detection of microaneurysms using stockwell transform and statistical features," *IET Image Processing*, vol. 13, no. 8, pp. 1341–1348, 2019.

[68] D. Jeba Derwin, S. Tamil Selvi, O. Jeba Singh, and B. Priestly Shan, "A novel automated system of discriminating microaneurysms in fundus images," *Biomedical Signal Processing and Control*, vol. 58, p. 101839, 2020.

[69] M. M. Fraz, P. Remagnino, A. Hoppe, B.Uyyanonvara, A. R. Rudnicka, C. G. Owen, and S. A. Barman, "Blood vessel segmentation methodologies in retinal images — A survey," *Computer Methods and Programs in Biomedicine*, vol. 108, pp. 407–433, 2012.

[70] C. Sinthanayothin, J. Boyce, H. Cook, and T. Williamson, "Automated local-isation of the optic disc, fovea, and retinal blood vessels from digital colour fundus images," *British Journal of Ophthalmology*, vol. 83, p. 902–910, 1999.

[71] M. Niemeijer, J.J.Staal, B. Van-Ginneken, M. Loog, and M. Abramoff, "Comparative study of retinal vessel segmentation methods on a new publicly available database," *in: J.M. Fitzpatrick, M. Sonka (Eds.)SPIE Medical Imaging. SPIE*, vol. 24, p. 648–656, 2004.

[72] J. Staal, M.D.Abramoff, M. Niemeijer, M. Viergever, and B. Van-Ginneken, "Ridge-based vessel segmentation in color images of the retina.," *IEEE Transactions on Medical Imaging*, vol. 23, p. 501–509, 2004.

[73] J. Soares, J. Leandro, R. Cesar, H. Jelinek, and M. Cree, "Retinal vessel segmentation using the 2-d gabor wavelet and supervised classification," *IEEE Transactions on Medical Imaging*, vol. 25, p. 1214–1222, 2006.

[74] E. Ricci and R. Perfetti, "Retinal blood vessel segmentation using line operators and support vector classification," *IEEE Transactions on Medical Imaging*, vol. 26, pp. 1357–1365, 2007.

[75] C. Lupascu, D. Tegolo, and E. Trucco, "FABC: retinal vessel segmentation using adaboost," *IEEE Transactions on Information Technology in Biomedicine*, vol. 14, p. 1267–1274, 2010.

[76] X. You, Q. Peng, Y. Yuan, Y. M.Cheung, and J. Lei, "Segmentation of retinal blood vessels using the radial projection and semi-supervised approach," *Pattern Recognition*, vol. 44, p. 2314–2324, 2011.

[77] D. Marin, A. Aquino, M. Gegundez-Arias, and J. Bravo, "A new supervised method for blood vessel segmentation in retinal images by using gray-level and moment invariants-based feature," *IEEE Transactions on Medical Imaging*, vol. 30, pp. 146–158, 2011.

[78] M. M. Fraz, P. Remagnino, A. Hoppe, B. Uyyanonvara, A. R. Rudnicka, C. G. Owen, and S. A. Barman, "An ensemble classification-based approach applied to retinal blood vessel segmentation," *IEEE Transactions on Biomedical Engineering*, vol. 59, pp. 2538–2548, 2012.

[79] R. Vega, G. Sanchez-Ante, L. E. Falcon-Morales, H. Sossa, and E. Guevara, "Retinal vessel extraction using lattice neural networks with dendritic processing," *Computers in Biology and Medicine*, vol. 58, pp. 20–30, 2015.

[80] S. W. Franklin and S. E. Rajan, "Retinal vessel segmentation employing ann technique by gabor and moment invariants-based features," *Applied Soft Computing*, vol. 22, pp. 94–100, 2014.

[81] S. Roychowdhury, D. D. Koozekanani, and K. K. Parhi, "Blood vessel segmentation of fundus images by major vessel extraction and subimage classification," *IEEE Journal of Biomedical and Health Informatics*, vol. 19, pp. 1118–1128, 2015.

[82] C. Zhu, B. Zou, R. Zhao, J. Cui, X. Duan, Z. Chen, and Y. Liang, "Retinal vessel segmentation in colour fundus images using extreme learning machine," *Computerized Medical Imaging and Graphics*, vol. 55, pp. 68–77, 2017.

[83] S. Wang, Y. Yin, G. Cao, B. Wei, Y. Zheng, and G. Yang, "Hierarchical retinal blood vessel segmentation based on feature and ensemble learning," *Neurocomputing*, vol. 149, pp. 708–717, 2015.

[84] H. Fu, Y. Xu, D. W. K. Wong, and J. Liu, "Retinal vessel segmentation via deep learning network and fully-connected conditional random fields," in *2016 IEEE 13th International Symposium on Biomedical Imaging (ISBI)*, pp. 698–701, 2016.

[85] K. Hu, Z. Zhang, X. Niu, Y. Zhang, C. Cao, F. Xiao, and X. Gao, "Retinal vessel segmentation of color fundus images using multiscale convolutional neural network with an improved cross-entropy loss function," *Neurocomputing*, vol. 309, pp. 179–191, 2018.

[86] Y. Jiang, N. Tan, T. Peng, and H. Zhang, "Retinal vessels segmentation based on dilated multi-scale convolutional neural network," *IEEE Access*, vol. 7, pp. 76342–76352, 2019.

[87] P. Liskowski and K. Krawiec, "Segmenting retinal blood vessels with deep neural networks," *IEEE Transactions on Medical Imaging*, vol. 35, no. 11, pp. 2369–2380, 2016.

[88] J. Long, E. Shelhamer, and T. Darrell, "Fully convolutional networks for semantic segmentation," in *2015 IEEE Conference on Computer Vision and Pattern Recognition (CVPR)*, pp. 3431–3440, 2015.

[89] A. Dasgupta and S. Singh, "A fully convolutional neural network based structured prediction approach towards the retinal vessel segmentation," in *2017 IEEE 14th International Symposium on Biomedical Imaging (ISBI 2017)*, pp. 248–251, 2017.

[90] İbrahim Atli and O. S. Gedik, "Sine-net: A fully convolutional deep learning architecture for retinal blood vessel segmentation," *Engineering Science and Technology, an International Journal*, 2020.

[91] S. Feng, Z. Zhuo, D. Pan, and Q. Tian, "Ccnet: A cross-connected convolutional network for segmenting retinal vessels using multi-scale features," *Neurocomputing*, vol. 392, pp. 268–276, 2020.

[92] Z. Jiang, H. Zhang, Y. Wang, and S.-B. Ko, "Retinal blood vessel segmentation using fully convolutional network with transfer learning," *Computerized Medical Imaging and Graphics*, vol. 68, pp. 1–15, 2018.

[93] O. Ronneberger, P. Fischer, and T. Brox, "U-net: Convolutional networks for biomedical image segmentation," in *Medical Image Computing and Computer-Assisted Intervention – MICCAI 2015*, pp. 234–241, Springer International Publishing, 2015.

[94] Q. Jin, Z. Meng, T. D. Pham, Q. Chen, L. Wei, and R. Su, "Dunet: A deformable network for retinal vessel segmentation," *Knowledge-Based Systems*, vol. 178, pp. 149–162, 2019.

[95] C. Guo, M. Szemenyei, Y. Yi, W. Zhou, and H. Bian, "Residual spatial attention network for retinal vessel segmentation," in *Neural Information Processing*, pp. 509–519, 2020.

[96] M. Z. Alom, M. Hasan, C. Yakopcic, T. Taha, and V. Asari, "Recurrent residual convolutional neural network based on U-net (R2U-net) for medical image segmentation," *Journal of Medical Imaging*, 02 2018.

[97] R. Azad, M. Asadi-Aghbolaghi, M. Fathy, and S. Escalera, "Bi-directional convlstm u-net with densley connected convolutions," in *2019 IEEE/CVF International Conference on Computer Vision Workshop (ICCVW)*, pp. 406–415, 2019.

[98] X. Guo, C. Chen, Y. Lu, K. Meng, H. Chen, K. Zhou, Z. Wang, and R. Xiao, "Retinal vessel segmentation combined with generative adversarial networks and dense u-net," *IEEE Access*, vol. 8, pp. 194551–194560, 2020.

[99] M. Niemeijer, B. van Ginneken, M. J. Cree, A. Mizutani, G. Quellec, C. I. Sanchez, B. Zhang, R. Hornero, M. Lamard, C. Muramatsu, X. Wu, G. Cazuguel, J. You, A. Mayo, Q. Li, Y. Hatanaka, B. Cochener, C. Roux, F. Karray, M. Garcia, H. Fujita, and M. D. Abramoff, "Retinopathy online challenge: Automatic detection of microaneurysms in digital color fundus photographs," *IEEE Transactions on Medical Imaging*, vol. 29, pp. 185–195, Jan 2010.

[100] T. Kauppi, V. Kalesnykiene, J.-K. Kamarainen, L. Lensu, I. Sorri, H. Uusitalo, H. Kälviäinen, and J. Pietilä, "Diaretdb0: Evaluation database and methodology for diabetic retinopathy algorithms," 2007.

[101] T. Kauppi, V. Kalesnykiene, J.-K. Kamarainen, L. Lensu, I. Sorri, A. Raninen, R. Voutilainen, H. Uusitalo, H. Kälviäinen, and J. Pietilä, "Diaretdb1 diabetic retinopathy database and evaluation protocol," in *Proc. Medical Image Understanding and Analysis (MIUA)*, vol. 2007, 01 2007.

[102] A. D. Hoover, V. Kouznetsova, and M. Goldbaum, "Locating blood vessels in retinal images by piecewise threshold probing of a matched filter response," *IEEE Transactions on Medical Imaging*, vol. 19, pp. 203–210, 2000.

[103] E. Decencière, G. Cazuguel, X. Zhang, G. Thibault, J.-C. Klein, F. Meyer, B. Marcotegui, G. Quellec, M. Lamard, R. Danno, D. Elie, P. Massin, Z. Viktor, A. Erginay, B. Laÿ, and A. Chabouis, "Teleophta: Machine learning and image processing methods for teleophthalmology," *IRBM*, vol. 34, no. 2, pp. 196–203, 2013.

[104] EyePACS, "Kaggle diabetic retinopathy detection database," *Available: https://www.kaggle.com/c/diabetic-retinopathy-detection*, 2015.

[105] L. Giancardo, F. Meriaudeau, T. P. Karnowski, Y. Li, S. Garg, K. W. Tobin, and E. Chaum, "Exudate-based diabetic macular edema detection in fundus images using publicly available datasets," *Medical Image Analysis*, vol. 16, no. 1, pp. 216–226, 2012.

[106] E. Decencière, X. Zhang, G. Cazuguel, B. Lay, B. Cochener, C. Trone, P. Gain, R. Ordonez, P. Massin, A. Erginay, B. Charton, and J.-C. Klein, "Feedback on a publicly distributed image database: The MESSIDOR Database," *Image Analysis Stereology*, vol. 33, no. 3, 2014.

[107] J. Sivaswamy, S. Krishnadas, G. D. Joshi, M. Jain, and A. U. S. Tabish, "Drishti-gs: Retinal image dataset for optic nerve head (onh) segmentation," in *2014 IEEE 11th International Symposium on Biomedical Imaging (ISBI)*, pp. 53–56, IEEE, 2014.

[108] P. Porwal, S. Pachade, R. Kamble, M. Kokare, G. Deshmukh, V. Sahasrabuddhe, and F. Meriaudeau, "Indian diabetic retinopathy image dataset (IDRiD)," *IEEE Dataport*, 2018.

[109] B. Al-Diri, A. Hunter, D. Steel, M. Habib, T. Hudaib, and S. Berry, "Review-a reference data set for retinal vessel profiles," in *2008 30th Annual International Conference of the IEEE Engineering in Medicine and Biology Society*, pp. 2262–2265, IEEE, 2008.

[110] E. J. Carmona, M. Rincón, J. García-Feijoó, and J. M. Martínez-de-la Casa, "Identification of the optic nerve head with genetic algorithms," *Artificial Intelligence in Medicine*, vol. 43, no. 3, pp. 243–259, 2008.

[111] A. Almazroa, S. Alodhayb, E. Osman, E. Ramadan, M. Hummadi, M. Dlaim, M. Alkatee, K. Raahemifar, and V. Lakshminarayanan, "Retinal fundus images for glaucoma analysis: the riga dataset," in *Medical Imaging 2018: Imaging Informatics for Healthcare, Research, and Applications*, vol. 10579, p. 105790B, International Society for Optics and Photonics, 2018.

[112] F. Fumero, S. Alayón, J. L. Sanchez, J. Sigut, and M. Gonzalez-Hernandez, "Rim-one: An open retinal image database for optic nerve evaluation," in *2011 24th international symposium on computer-based medical systems (CBMS)*, pp. 1–6, IEEE, 2011.

[113] T. Köhler, A. Budai, M. F. Kraus, J. Odstrčilik, G. Michelson, and J. Horneg-ger, "Automatic no-reference quality assessment for retinal fundus images using vessel segmentation," in *Proceedings of the 26th IEEE International Symposium on Computer-Based Medical Systems*, pp. 95–100, IEEE, 2013.

[114] VARPA, "The vicvar database," *Available: http://www.varpa.es/vicvar.html*, 2014.

[115] E. Grisan, M. Foracchia, A. Ruggeri, *et al.*, "A novel method for the au-tomatic grading of retinal vessel tortuosity," *IEEE Transactions on Medical Imaging*, vol. 27, no. 3, pp. 310–319, 2008.

[116] ARIA, "Retinal image archive," *http://www.eyecharity.com*, Last accessed on 15th Feruary 2015.

[117] M. Niemeijer, X. Xu, A. V. Dumitrescu, P. Gupta, B. Van Ginneken, J. C. Folk, and M. D. Abramoff, "Automated measurement of the arteriolar-to-venular width ratio in digital color fundus photographs," *IEEE Transactions on Medical Imaging*, vol. 30, no. 11, pp. 1941–1950, 2011.

[118] R. Anderson, C. Tiago, F. J. Herbert, G. Siome, and W. Jacques, "Points of interest and visual dictionaries for automatic retinal lesion detection," *IEEE Transaction on Biomedical Engineering,*, vol. 59, no. 8, pp. 2244–2253, 2012.

[119] A. M.U. and A. S. Khan, "Automated detection of dark and bright lesions in retinal images for early detection of diabetic retinopathy," *Journal of Medical Systems*, vol. 36, pp. 3151–3162, 2012.

[120] A. Sopharak, B. Uyyanonvara, and S. Barman, "Simple hybrid method for fine microaneurysm detection from non-dilated diabetic retinopathy retinal images," *Computerized Medical Imaging and Graphics*, vol. 37, pp. 394–402, 2013.

[121] R. C. Gonzalez, R. E. Woods, and S. L. Eddins, *Digital Image Processing Using MATLAB*. 2nd ed. McGraw Hill Education, 2010.

[122] M. Luo, M. Yu-Fei, and Z. Hong-Jiang, "A spatial constrained k-means approach to image segmentation," *Fourth International Conference on Information, Communications and Signal Processing.*, vol. 2, pp. 738–742, 2003.

[123] X. Zhu, R. M. Rangayyan, and L. E. Anna, *Automated Image Detection of RETINAL PATHOLOGY*. London Newyork: CRC Press, 2011.

[124] M. D. Abramoff, M. Niemeijer, S. Maria, M. A. Viergever, R. S. R., and B. V. Ginneken, "Evaluation of a system for automatic detection of diabetic retinopathy from color fundus photographs in a large population of patients with diabetes," *Journal of Diabetes Care*, vol. 31, pp. 193–198, 2008.

[125] M.-K. Hu, "Visual pattern recognition by moment invariants," *IRE Trans. Information Theory*, vol. 8, pp. 179–187, 1962.

[126] A. Khotanzad and Y. H. Hong, "Invariant image recognition by zernike moments," *IEEE Transactions on Pattern Analysis and Machine Intelligence*, vol. 12, no. 5, pp. 489–497, 1990.

[127] A. Tahmasbi, F. Saki, and S. B. Shokouhi, "Classification of benign and malignant masses based on zernike moments," *Computers in Biology and Medicine*, vol. 41, no. 8, pp. 726–735, 2011.

[128] C. Seiffert, T. M. Khoshgoftaar, J. Van Hulse, and A. Napolitano, "Rusboost: A hybrid approach to alleviating class imbalance," *IEEE Transactions on Systems, Man, and Cybernetics - Part A: Systems and Humans*, vol. 40, no. 1, pp. 185–197, 2010.

[129] Y. Freund and R. E. Schapire, "Experiments with a new boosting algorithm," in *Proceedings of the Thirteenth International Conference on International Conference on Machine Learning*, p. 148–156, 1996.

[130] M. F. Mohammed and C. P. Lim, "An enhanced fuzzy min—max neural network for pattern classification," *IEEE Transactions on Neural Networks and Learning Systems*, vol. 26, pp. 417–429, 2015.

[131] M. H. Asghari and B. Jalali, "Edge detection in digital images using dispersive phase stretch transform," *International Journal of Biomedical Imaging*, pp. 1–7, 2015.

[132] P. Kovesi, "Image features from phase congruency," *Videre: A Journal of Computer Vision Research. MIT Press*, vol. 1, pp. 1–27, 1999.

[133] A. F. Frangi, W. J. Niessen, K. L. Vincken, and M. A. Viergever, "Multiscale vessel enhancement filtering," *Medical Image Computing and Computer Assisted Intervention MICCAI-98*, pp. 130–137, 1998.

[134] B. Gabrys and A. Bargiela, "General fuzzy min-max neural network for clustering and classification," *IEEE Transactions on Neural Networks*, vol. 11, p. 769–783, 2000.

[135] P. K. Simpson, "Fuzzy min-max neural networks-i classification," *IEEE Transactions on Neural Networks*, vol. 3, pp. 776–786, 1992.

[136] S. Wang, Y. Yin, G. Cao, B. Wei, Y. Zheng, and G. Yang, "Hierarchical retinal blood vessel segmentation based on feature and ensemble learning," *Neurocomputing*, vol. 149, pp. 708–717, 2015.

[137] S. Ruder, "Transfer Learning - Machine Learning's Next Frontier." http://ruder.io/transfer-learning/, 2017.

[138] S. Woo, J. Park, J.-Y. Lee, and I. S. Kweon, "Cbam: Convolutional block attention module," in *Computer Vision – ECCV 2018*, pp. 3–19, 2018.

[139] S. J. Pan and Q. Yang, "A survey on transfer learning," *IEEE Transactions on Knowledge and Data Engineering*, vol. 22, no. 10, pp. 1345–1359, 2010.

[140] Q. Li, B. Feng, L. Xie, P. Liang, H. Zhang, and T. Wang, "A cross-modality learning approach for vessel segmentation in retinal images," *IEEE Transactions on Medical Imaging*, vol. 35, no. 1, pp. 109–118, 2016.

[141] J. Mo and L. Zhang, "Multi-level deep supervised networks for retinal vessel segmentation," *International Journal of Computer Assisted Radiology and Surgery volume*, vol. 12, pp. 2181–2193, 2017.

[142] Z. Yan, X. Yang, and K. T. Cheng, "Joint segment-level and pixel-wise losses for deep learning based retinal vessel segmentation," *IEEE Transactions on Biomedical Engineering*, vol. 65, no. 9, pp. 1912–1923, 2018.

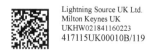